patrick
HOLFORD

The Feel Good Factor

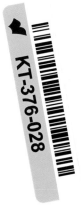

'In my experience this approach works far better than medication. It is the future of an enlightened approach to psychiatry.'

Dr Hyla Cass, psychiatrist and co-author of *Natural Highs*

'This book is a gem. As a psychiatrist, it has made simple the natural alternative to the conventional mainstream approaches to mental illness across the board. I would wholeheartedly recommend it, particularly to all working in the mental health field and generally to all concerned with their mental health.'

Dr Shauki Mahomed, psychiatrist

'My mood is great, it's easier to get up in the mornings and I have even joined a gym!'

Hannah, describing how she felt after three months of following a supplement programme and dietary advice. She had previously suffered from depression for seven years

'I feel much better. I'm very busy right now, and in the past I'd feel overwhelmed and not able to cope, both mentally and physically, but now I feel great. My mood is very positive – no panic or depression. I feel buoyant, energetic and enthusiastic.'

Amanda-Jane, two months after beginning her supplement and diet regime

'I've been trying to feel like this for 25 years – I'm over the moon!'

Gabrielle, who had suffered from extreme lethargy and mood swings for decades. She was found to have a huge deficiency in vitamin D with low to borderline essential fats and was also chronically low in serotonin, the brain's mood-boosting neurotransmitter. She started a supplement programme to correct the deficiencies and almost immediately began to feel an improvement in her symptoms

'It's made a substantial difference. I feel much more balanced and have a much more positive, rather than negative, outlook on life.'

Holly, who had been plagued with anxiety, low moods and indecisiveness for years. Her main problem, it turned out, was vitamin D deficiency

patrick
HOLFORD

The Feel Good Factor

piatkus

PIATKUS

First published in Great Britain in 2010 by Piatkus
Copyright © Patrick Holford 2010
The moral right of the author has been asserted.

A CIP catalogue record for this book
is available from the British Library.

ISBN 978-0-7499-5316-4

Typeset in 11.5/15pt Minion by Phoenix Photosetting, Chatham, Kent
Printed and bound in Great Britain by CPI Mackays, Chatham, ME5 8TD

Papers used by Piatkus are natural, renewable and recyclable
products sourced from well-managed forests and certified
in accordance with the rules of the Forest Stewardship Council.

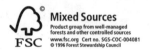

Mixed Sources
Product group from well-managed
forests and other controlled sources
www.fsc.org Cert no. SGS-COC-004081
© 1996 Forest Stewardship Council
FSC

Piatkus
An imprint of
Little, Brown Book Group
100 Victoria Embankment
London EC4Y 0DY

An Hachette UK Company
www.hachette.co.uk

www.piatkus.co.uk

ABOUT THE AUTHOR

Patrick Holford BSc, DipION, FBANT, NTCRP is a leading spokesman on nutrition in the media, specialising in the field of mental health. He is the author of over 30 books, translated into over 20 languages and selling over a million copies worldwide, including *The Optimum Nutrition Bible, The Low GL-Diet Bible, Optimum Nutrition for the Mind* and *The Alzheimer's Prevention Plan.*

Patrick started his academic career in the field of psychology. He then became a student of two of the leading pioneers in nutrition medicine and psychiatry – the late Dr Carl Pfeiffer and Dr Abram Hoffer. In 1984 he founded the Institute for Optimum Nutrition (ION), an independent educational charity, with his mentor, twice Nobel Prize winner Dr Linus Pauling, as patron. ION has been researching and helping to define what it means to be optimally nourished for the past 25 years and is one of the most respected educational establishments for training nutritional therapists. At ION he was involved in groundbreaking research showing that multivitamins can increase children's IQ scores – the subject of a *Horizon* TV documentary in the 1980s. He was one of the first promoters of the importance of zinc, antioxidants, essential fats, low-GL diets and homocysteine-lowering B vitamins and their importance in mental health and Alzheimer's disease prevention.

Patrick is director of the Food for the Brain Foundation and director of the Brain Bio Centre, the Foundation's treatment centre that specialises in helping those with mental issues ranging from depression to schizophrenia. He is an honorary fellow of the British Association of Nutritional Therapy, as well as a member of the Nutrition Therapy Council.

BY THE SAME AUTHOR

100% Health

500 Top Health and Nutrition Questions Answered

Balancing Hormones Naturally (with Kate Neil)

Beat Stress and Fatigue

Boost Your Immune System (with Jennifer Meek)

Food GLorious Food (with Fiona McDonald Joyce)

Hidden Food Allergies (with Dr James Braly)

How to Quit Without Feeling S**t (with David Miller and Dr James Braly)

Improve Your Digestion

Natural Highs (with Dr Hyla Cass)

Optimum Nutrition Before, During and After Pregnancy (with Susannah Lawson)

Optimum Nutrition for the Mind

Optimum Nutrition for Your Child (with Deborah Colson)

Optimum Nutrition Made Easy

Say No to Arthritis

Say No to Cancer

Say No to Heart Disease

Six Weeks to Superhealth

Smart Food for Smart Kids (with Fiona McDonald Joyce)

Solve Your Skin Problems (with Natalie Savona)

The 10 Secrets of 100% Healthy People

The Alzheimer's Prevention Plan (with Shane Heaton and Deborah Colson)

The H Factor (with Dr James Braly)

The Holford 9-day Liver Detox (with Fiona McDonald Joyce)

The Holford Diet GL Counter

The Little Book of Optimum Nutrition

The Low-GL Diet Bible

The Low-GL Diet Cookbook (with Fiona McDonald Joyce)

The Optimum Nutrition Bible

The Optimum Nutrition Cookbook (with Judy Ridgway)

The Perfect Pregnancy Cookbook (with Fiona McDonald Joyce)

CONTENTS

ACKNOWLEDGEMENTS

For the original inspiration to explore this rich seam of nutrition, I am deeply indebted to the late Dr Carl Pfeiffer and Dr Abram Hoffer, the true pioneers of 'orthomolecular' psychiatry and the power of nutrition to promote mental health. I owe a debt of gratitude to all the team at the Brain Bio Centre, our psychiatrists and clinical nutritionists, Lorraine Perretta and Deborah Colson, and the clinic manager Bronia Novak, who tirelessly help people find their way back to living a full and rewarding life.

On the psychological front, I'd like to thank Dr Shauki Mahomed, Dr Beverly Feinberg Moss and Nan Beecher-Moore for their guidance and insight. I'd also like to thank all those who have shared their stories of transformation in the hope that they will motivate others.

I'd also like to thank Sharon Watson for her help with the research, Jillian Stewart and Jan Cutler for their help with editing, and Gill Bailey and Tim Whiting at Piatkus for their support and encouragement to publish this book and get it to as many people as possible.

Disclaimer

Although all the nutrients and dietary changes referred to in this book have been proven safe, those seeking help for specific medical conditions are advised to consult a qualified nutrition therapist, clinical nutritionist, doctor or equivalent health professional. The recommendations given in this book are solely intended as education and information, and should not be taken as medical advice. Neither the author nor the publisher accept liability for readers who choose to self-prescribe.

All supplements should be kept out of reach of infants and young children.

If you are seeing a psychotherapist or you are on medication

Under supervision of a doctor or psychiatrist, the recommendations in this book don't replace those received from your health-care practitioners; however, much of the advice in this book can be followed alongside other approaches. When there are contraindications between specific nutritional supplements and medication, I will make this clear. If you are suffering from a chronic mental health problem and would like to pursue a nutritional approach with professional guidance, you can refer yourself, or be referred by your doctor, to our Brain Bio Centre (see Resources). We work with people from all over the world, sometimes partnering with local nutritional therapists who can continue your supervised support. The first step to take is to read this book.

Guide to Abbreviations, Measures and References

Vitamins

1 gram (g) = 1,000 milligrams (mg) = 1,000,000 micrograms (mcg, also written as μg)

Most vitamins are measured in milligrams or micrograms. Vitamins A, D and E used to be measured in International Units (iu), a measurement designed to standardise the various forms of these vitamins, which have different potencies.

6mcg of beta-carotene, the vegetable precursor of vitamin A is, on average, converted into 1mcg of retinol, the animal form of vitamin A. So, 6mcg of beta-carotene is called 1mcgRE (RE stands for retinol equivalent). Throughout this book beta-carotene is referred to in mcgRE.

1mcg of retinol (1mcgRE) = 3.3iu of vitamin A
1mcgRE of beta-carotene = 6mcg of beta-carotene
100iu of vitamin D = 2.5mcg
100iu of vitamin E = 67mg
1 pound (lb) = 16 ounces (oz)
2.2lb = 1 kilogram (kg)
1 pint = 0.6 litres
1.76 pints = 1 litre
In this book 'calories' means kilocalories (kcals)

References and further reading

In each part of the book, you'll find numbered references. These refer to research papers listed in the References section on page 224, and are there for readers who want to study this subject in depth. On pages 242–44 you will find a list of the best books to read to enable you to dig deeper into the topics covered. You will also find that many of the topics touched on in this book are covered in detail in feature articles available at www.patrickholford.com. If you want to stay up to date with all that is new and exciting in this field, I recommend you subscribe to my *100% Health* newsletter, details of which are on the website www.patrickholford.com.

INTRODUCTION

Whether you just feel low and unmotivated, or you suffer from severe depression or constant anxiety, this book will help you to regain the Feel Good Factor. It might seem unlikely if you're currently feeling down but you *can* wake up full of energy, in a good mood and with motivation for the day – that's the Feel Good Factor and I believe it is our natural state and the right of everyone. No matter how you feel at present, it is within your power to deal with the unexpected events of life without crumbling or feeling down, anxious, irritable and unable to sleep.

The reason I say this with confidence is that I've seen hundreds of people who have come to our Brain Bio Centre in Richmond, near London, often seriously depressed and struggling with mental health issues, who have left feeling not just in control but positively great.

'It's made a substantial difference. I feel much more balanced and have a much more positive, rather than negative, outlook on life,' says Holly, who had been plagued with anxiety, low moods and indecisiveness for years. Her main problem, it turned out, was vitamin D deficiency.

'I've been trying to feel like this for 25 years – I'm over the moon!' said Gabrielle, who had suffered from extreme lethargy and mood swings for decades. She was also chronically low in serotonin, the brain's mood-boosting neurotransmitter, easily boosted by a simple amino acid supplement.

A journalist who had suffered from depression rang me, not for an interview but simply to say thank you. She had followed the advice that I give in this book and had come out of her depression not in weeks or days but in hours. In her case the mineral chromium made all the difference. Another journalist, who had suffered bouts of disabling depression and sought help at the Brain Bio Centre, said this, one week after starting the nutritional regime: 'I woke up and I knew immediately that the black mood had lifted. It seemed, to my distinct surprise, that I might be better. Despite my lack of faith, a minor miracle had happened.'

Of course, simply following the advice in this book doesn't mean you'll never experience emotions such as sadness, anger or fear again. Emotions are there to show us something, and to be 'e-moted' – in other words, expressed and moved through. They do not need to be residual and debilitating. We all go through bad patches due to changes, traumas and losses in life. Your ability to learn and move through these phases and bounce back into life with renewed enthusiasm has as much to do with recharging the brain and body's biochemistry as it does with resolving psychological issues, as I am going to show you.

The mind–body chemistry connection

If there is one thing that is emerging in the modern-day understanding of psychological health it is the interplay between our thoughts, feelings and physical sensations and our body's biochemistry. What we think changes how we feel, and vice versa. Feelings are always accompanied by physical sensations. But all of these are also associated with corresponding changes in our internal biochemistry. Biochemical changes also affect how we feel and think. For example, when 15 women in a trial at Oxford University were given a diet devoid of the amino acid tryptophan – from which your brain makes the feel-good chemical serotonin – ten out of 15 started feeling more depressed within seven hours. That's how close the link is between what you eat and how you feel.

To exacerbate matters, the worse you feel the more you turn to comfort foods, which are high in sugar, and look for ways to numb the pain, perhaps by eating too much or drinking too much alcohol. This, in turn, depletes your energy to deal with life's obstacles, making you feel more and more tired and low. It is all one great big web of factors, from the circumstances of your life to the food on your plate, and how you react to the thoughts and feelings in between. By unravelling this web I'm going to show you how to take control of how you feel.

Knowing this, one of the obvious deficits of conventional psychiatry is that most diagnoses are based solely on questionnaires centred on psychological symptoms, and the majority of diagnosed problems, from insomnia to depression, are then treated with chemical drugs – hopefully alongside psychotherapy. At the Brain Bio Centre, however, we test for biochemical imbalances, then correct them with *nutrients*, not drugs. They are more effective, less expensive and don't have undesirable side effects. These nutrients, which are already present in the body, will work together to help 'tune up' your system and pave the way for feeling good while avoiding the use of man-made drugs with their often worrying side effects. In a sense, psychotherapeutic approaches are like teaching you to drive better, but your car may need a tune-up to make it easier to drive. That's where nutrition comes in.

Do antidepressants do more harm than good?

Conventional opinion would say that the purpose of medication such as antidepressant drugs is to get you back on the road. However, as you'll see in Chapter 4, antidepressant drugs have a lousy track record when it comes to success, and have a plethora of side effects that can often leave you worse off than when you started. An analysis of six large studies published in the *Journal of the American Medical Association* found that for people with mild or moderate depression, which accounts for the vast majority of people with diagnosed depression, antidepressants are really no better than a placebo.[1] To quote the study, 'The magnitude of benefit of antidepressant medication compared with placebo ... may be minimal or nonexistent, on average, in patients with mild or moderate symptoms.' A recent report on all treatments for depression from the UK's National Institute for Health and Clinical Excellence (NICE) agrees, 'There is little clinically important difference between antidepressants and placebo for mild depression.'[2]

Even more concerning are the side effects. Prozac (fluoxetine), for example, has 45 listed side effects. Prozac and another commonly prescribed antidepressant, Seroxat (paroxetine), show clear evidence of agitation leading to potential aggressive and suicidal behaviour in as many as a quarter of patients in a number of clinical trials. But don't think that newer antidepressants are any better. They are not. (I examine this issue in detail in Chapter 4.)

A different approach

Nutritional therapy, on the other hand, has nothing but benefits. As you'll discover in this book, there is evidence of the effectiveness of many nutritional approaches – things that are easy for you to do right now without any downsides. Sadly, few doctors are aware of them, or have received training in nutritional therapy or experienced first hand the kind of effects that it can deliver. In fact, many doctors have an inbuilt suspicion of nutritional medicine, largely due to brainwashing by the pharmaceutical industry.

Depression is big business

Mind-altering prescription drugs such as antidepressants are exceedingly big business, bringing in over $30 billion a year. In America, even by 2005, 27 million people – that's one in ten – had been prescribed them. And today, who knows how many are on medication?[3] The numbers keep going up and up, and so does the money. And that amount of money buys a lot of 'air time' in medical journals, and funding for medical training and post-graduate conferences, as well as keeping doctors in the dark about safer and more effective alternatives.

How I discovered a different path

I am no stranger to low moods. I am sure there are some people who nearly always feel good and roll with the punches of life, but I suspect that most of us have times when we feel low, ranging from just feeling flat to downright depressed.

As a child I witnessed a family member struggle with depression, having breakdowns and trying medication and psychotherapy along the way. It inspired me to study psychology, and I was ever hopeful that somewhere in the world of psychotherapy lay the answers to the meaning of life and how to feel good almost all the time. I tried all sorts of different approaches, from meditation techniques to different psychotherapeutic approaches and cathartic emotional work – you name it, I tried it. I also explored what happens in the brain, and in the brain's chemistry, when we feel good and when we don't and how it is possible to manipulate this, with drugs but also with nutrients. The nutrients I explored were naturally occurring substances from which our brain's feel-good chemicals are actually made.

The origins of nutritional psychiatry

This led me into the world of nutritional therapy as opposed to drug therapy and, to my amazement, the results were not only more effective for many types of mental-health problems but also less dangerous with virtually no side effects. Instead, there were many other positive health benefits.

I became a student in the late 1970s and early 1980s of two of the leading pioneers in mental health and nutrition, Dr Carl Pfeiffer and Dr Abram Hoffer, who pioneered the treatment of schizophrenia in Canada using nutritional medicine, and who helped thousands of people to recover. Hoffer also published several hundred research papers, including the first ever 'double blind' controlled trial in the history of psychiatry, showing that a high dose of niacin (vitamin B_3) was more effective than drugs for schizophrenia. The side effect of using niacin was that it also lowered cholesterol and it can now be prescribed by doctors for that very purpose.

I also became a student of the late Dr Linus Pauling, recipient of two Nobel Prizes and 48 PhDs. He pioneered the concept of 'orthomolecular' psychiatry: the science of giving the optimum (ortho) naturally occurring molecules (that is, nutrients) to restore mental health and energy. I called this 'optimum nutrition' and founded the Institute for Optimum Nutrition (ION) in 1984 to explore the role of nutrition in helping to prevent and reverse physical and mental health problems. More than a decade ago we set up a clinic called the Brain Bio Centre specifically to help those with mental-health problems, ranging from depression, anxiety and insomnia to schizophrenia and dementia. The Brain Bio Centre is the clinical division of the Food for the Brain Foundation (see www.foodforthebrain.org), our educational charity dedicated to informing people about the power nutrition has to improve how we feel.

Our team includes psychiatrists and nutritional therapists, guided by a board of scientific advisors – professors with expertise in various aspects of mental health. Thousands of people have sought help, and found it, by applying simple, scientifically proven principles that should be part of mainstream medicine but sadly remain excluded, due to an institutionalised suspicion of nutritional therapy in favour of drugs.

As you will see in this book, the results, proven in research and illustrated by the cases of people whose lives have been transformed, show that these approaches are not only often more effective than conventional medicine but they are also much better for you. You will be able to replicate these results by working through the advice I give you in the chapters that follow.

Why eating a 'well-balanced diet' is not enough

The stark truth is that most of us do not get all the nutrients we need from a so-called well-balanced diet. As you will see, if your system is out of balance, conceivably due to purely circumstantial stresses and traumas, the amount of certain nutrients you will need to reset your system to feeling good is far more than you can achieve just by eating more fish, fruit and vegetables.

For this reason, I focus more on the proven nutritional approaches to making you feel good. However, I also explain the important psychological approaches and lifestyle changes that work, giving you the necessary resources to find the help you need to regain your Feel Good Factor.

Think of your mental health as a deposit account. When it is depleted by traumas and stresses, by an unfulfilling job or relationship, when it is robbed of nutrients by eating refined and processed foods, and by too much caffeine, alcohol and sugar, and when it is further depleted by various medications, you become 'overdrawn' and unable to find your own natural Feel Good Factor. I'm going to show you how to put money back into your mental health deposit account.

The purpose of this book is to get you back to feeling good and to show you how to stay there.

How to use this book

Part 1 starts with a detailed questionnaire that assesses your mood. This 'mood check' becomes your own way to measure what makes the biggest difference to how you feel as you go through the book putting into action the various suggestions I make. I then familiarise you with the different ways to improve your mental health, and explain why antidepressants are rarely the answer. This part of the book will improve your understanding of the 'science' of feeling good but it will also get you started on the road to feeling great by suggesting changes you can make right now to improve psychological factors, your lifestyle and your nutritional status.

Part 2 outlines my top ten proven ways to improve your mood. Each key factor in Part 2 contains a questionnaire, some with back-up home tests, to help you find out which factors are most important for *you*, because we are all different. This section really gets to the heart of what you can do to help yourself.

In Part 3 you'll find out how to put together your own Feel Good Factor regime including your best mood-boosting diet, supplement and lifestyle programme with all the practical information you need to be successful.

Wishing you the best of health and happiness,

Patrick Holford

Part One

THE ANATOMY OF FEELING GOOD

In this part you'll discover the essential steps that set you up for feeling good and why antidepressants aren't the answer. We'll be exploring both the chemistry and the psychology of mood and how your mind and body work together to create your experience of energy, motivation and mood. You'll also find out about the most effective natural remedies for restoring your joie de vivre.

Chapter 1

HOW HAPPY ARE YOU?

Do you leap out of bed in the morning, excited and looking forward to another day? If you had to rate yourself out of ten, where ten was feeling really good and enjoying life and 0 was rock bottom, where are you now? The chances are that you didn't score above 7, which is why you've bought this book. The goal of *The Feel Good Factor* is to help you get up there into the realm of feeling great most of the time.

First, let's explore the scale from 'happy and energised' to 'depressed and exhausted' in more detail, because this is going to be your yardstick for finding out which are the key factors that will help you feel good. 'Depression' is one of those words that can be used to describe a range of feelings: from how you feel when your football team loses, right through to utter despair, when life doesn't seem worth living. It can be a general feeling of being 'down' to being one of the most debilitating illnesses, leaving you incapable of working or having a stable relationship. Most people would not describe themselves as depressed, a label that has a certain stigma, but they also wouldn't describe themselves as feeling good.

Psychologists tell us that depressive feelings are often accompanied by anxiety, fear, anger, irritability, hopelessness and despair. An individual can easily become irritable and impatient with people and be prone to angry outbursts. But just how common are these feelings?

One in two people report often feeling low

On my website www.patrickholford.com there is an invitation to complete the 100% Health check-up. This is a free health questionnaire that takes about 20 minutes to complete. Each question has a scale of answers, usually from 'rarely' to 'frequently' and these are used to give you a score out of 100 per cent. Try scoring yourself now and see where you are (if you wish, you can also get a comprehensive report about your health and how to improve it).

Between 2000 and 2010, over 55,000 people completed the 100% Health questionnaire answering questions including these on mood:

Do you suffer from mood swings?	63%
Do you suffer from depression?	48%
Do you get anxious or tense easily?	66%
Do you get irritable easily?	66%
Do you generally feel apathetic and unmotivated?	58%
Have you had a drop in your motivation or drive?	62%
Do you have a low energy level?	81%
Do you easily become angry?	55%
Do you become impatient if people or things hold you up?	82%
Do you have difficulty sleeping or sleep restlessly?	55%

The percentage of people who answered 'frequently' or 'occasionally' is shown in the right-hand column. How do you compare? These percentages reflect how so many people feel. Some of us, when we feel really low, seek help, be it by speaking to our doctor or perhaps with the help of a counsellor or psychotherapist. But most of us put up with it, assuming that this is just life and that we should struggle on trying to make the circumstances of our lives better: a better partner, a better job, more money in the bank, a holiday in the sun…

Some of us, when times are really bad, will be put on medication, and often continue to take it even when we have felt much better for some time. Although the British have an inborn suspicion about taking antidepressants, the National Health Service in England alone spends over £250 million a year on them, dispensing 40 million prescriptions.[4] In America an estimated 10 per cent of people – that's 27 million – have been given antidepressants, which are now the most commonly prescribed class of medication in America.[5]

What determines your mood?

Why do we feel this way and how can we feel better? Often we have answers, reasons and excuses, and they are usually to do with something outside ourselves, such as: if I had better luck in life; if I could meet the right man/woman; if I had better friends/the right job/more money/more time to myself; if I lived somewhere different/knew what I wanted to do; or if I had a spiritual conviction… We sense that there is something 'out there' that would change how we feel inside.

Often, feeling down appears to be triggered by something 'bad' that has happened: a tragedy or something that changes our circumstances for the worse; a relationship goes pear-shaped, or perhaps someone close to you dies or you lose your health, your house, your partner, your money or your job, or you suffer humiliation or defeat. 'Feeling trapped and unable to control one's environment is one of the most common triggers for depression as well as one of the most commonly reported feelings of those that are depressed,' says Paul Gilbert, Professor of Clinical Psychology at the University of Derby in his book *Overcoming Depression*.

Something is missing

Whatever it is, there is a sense of 'lack' – something is missing. No doubt, better 'luck' would make a difference, but is happiness a matter of good fortune, of acquiring something? Or is it something you can create for yourself? After all, we all know people who seem to be happy most of the time despite circumstances much worse than our own. What is their secret? Or are they just simpler people with no ambition? If so, does that mean that someone like you can't be happy? Is a general state of happiness learned or inherited, a part of our genetic programming, a human right or a human illusion? No doubt you have already had these thoughts and tried different means to boost your mood. Perhaps you have read self-help books, or begun a new relationship, tried mind-altering substances such as Ecstasy or alcohol, practised exercises such as yoga or meditation, or even tried medication and counselling, but you've still not managed to improve your mood for long.

There's a veritable supermarket out there of different remedies, exercises, books and courses claiming to give you the Feel Good Factor. If you believe the ads, there are cars, drinks, snacks, perfumes, clothes, and even household cleaners, that promise to propel you into a state of virtual nirvana.

Why are some people happy but others sad?

In researching this book I've had access to questionnaires completed by 55,570 people, allowing me to see what's different about the diet, lifestyle and attitudes of those who wake up full of energy, with a good mood and motivation for the day. I've interviewed those who claim to have the best health and happiness to find their secret.

As well as learning from those with the best health and happiness scores, I've also learned from those at the other end of the scale – the thousands of people who have sought help at the Brain Bio Centre, our clinic near London, that specialises in nutritional approaches to mental health problems such as depression, anxiety and insomnia. And I've learned what has made them better, as you'll discover as you read through this book.

I've also investigated the many different avenues that are claimed to enhance mood, and I've examined the evidence to decipher those that truly work and why. This book is the result of some 30 years' exploration into the science of feeling good to help you discover the critical pieces that will help you jump several steps closer to feeling good most of the time.

In this chapter I list the factors that make us feel good, but first it's important to get a more comprehensive yardstick on where you are right now so that as you try out the different approaches you'll have some objective way of seeing what really makes a difference.

Check your mood

First, use the questionnaire opposite to find out where you fit on the continuum, from happy and content through prone to low moods, all the way down to clinically depressed. (No one but you will be looking at the answers, so be honest. If you prefer, write your answers on a sheet of paper.)

Questionnaire: Mood check

	Frequently	Occasionally	Rarely
1 Do you feel downhearted, depressed or sad?	☐	☐	☐
2 Do you feel worse in the morning?	☐	☐	☐
3 Do you have crying spells, or feel like crying?	☐	☐	☐
4 Do you have trouble falling asleep, or sleeping through the night?	☐	☐	☐
5 Is your appetite poor and are you losing weight without trying?	☐	☐	☐
6 Are you gaining weight or bingeing on sweet foods?	☐	☐	☐
7 Do you feel unattractive and unlovable?	☐	☐	☐
8 Do you prefer to be alone and shy away from social interaction?	☐	☐	☐
9 Do you feel fearful and easily panic about things?	☐	☐	☐
10 Do you feel anxious and nervous?	☐	☐	☐
11 Are you often tired?	☐	☐	☐
12 Do you easily become irritable or angry?	☐	☐	☐
13 Are you restless and unable to keep still?	☐	☐	☐
14 Do you feel hopeless about the future?	☐	☐	☐
15 Do you think you are letting people down, or have done in the past?	☐	☐	☐

	Frequently	Occasionally	Rarely
16 Is your mood affecting your work?	☐	☐	☐
17 Is it an effort to do the things you used to do with ease because of a lack of enthusiasm?	☐	☐	☐
18 Do you feel like you've slowed down?	☐	☐	☐
19 Do you find it difficult to make decisions?	☐	☐	☐
20 Do you worry about your health?	☐	☐	☐
21 Do you feel less enjoyment from activities that once gave you pleasure?	☐	☐	☐
22 Do you have less interest or desire for sex?	☐	☐	☐

Score 2 for each 'frequently' answer, 1 for 'occasionally' and 0 for 'rarely'.

Score

Below 5

You are normal. You appear to be positive, optimistic and able to roll with the punches. This book will give you clues on how to handle those occasions when things aren't going so well for you.

5–9

You have a mild case of the blues. Following the advice in this book will get you back on track.

10–15

You have a moderate case of the blues. As well as following the advice in this book you might benefit from some professional help, by seeing a psychotherapist and a nutritional therapist.

More than 15

You have plenty of symptoms of depression so, as well as reading this book, you will benefit from getting some professional help. I will explain how you can find it.

HAMILTON RATING SCALE FOR DEPRESSION

The mood check above is based on similar symptoms that are used in medical questionnaires designed to diagnose depression. One of the most widely used is called the Hamilton Rating Scale for Depression (Ham-D), which is also one of the most widely used tests to evaluate the effectiveness of different mood-boosting approaches; for example, antidepressant drugs or psychotherapy. If you are diagnosed with depression, it is usually on the basis of a scale such as the Ham-D, as it is often called. So, when we come to talk about studies that show, for example, a 30 per cent improvement in the Ham-D score, you'll have a good idea of what that means. I'll be using changes in the Ham-D scores as a reference to evaluate different approaches. You can also use the mood check above as a yardstick so that, as you try out the different factors that are given in Part 2 you can come back to this questionnaire and rate how you feel as a result.

Your symptoms will unlock your mood-boosting secrets

As you go through this book you'll see that many of these 'symptoms' – feeling tired, or anxious and edgy, or feeling low or unable to sleep and feel rested – relate to specific nutritional and biochemical imbalances, and you'll be able to identify, from your symptoms, which ones are most likely to help you.

For example:

If you feel tired a lot of the time, crave carbohydrates and are gaining weight, and can feel very oversensitive – for example, taking any form of criticism badly – these are symptoms that respond particularly well to balancing your blood sugar and taking the mineral chromium.

If you are prone to feeling low in the winter, picking up lots of infections and spending little time outdoors, you are probably lacking vitamin D.

If you feel generally low and unmotivated, have poor concentration and dry skin, and you rarely eat oily fish, there's a good chance that you're lacking in omega-3 essential fats.

If you are quite stressed, anxious and hyperactive, you can't sit still and you find it hard to relax and go to sleep, perhaps suffering from muscle cramps or restless legs, and if you rarely eat seeds and nuts and don't eat enough green vegetables, there's a good chance you are lacking in magnesium.

What those mood-boosters are

In Part 2 I'm going to explain in detail the most common biochemical and nutritional causes of feeling low, and the proven ways to boost how you feel. In a nutshell these are:

Blood sugar imbalances. These can be corrected by eating the right diet – one that has a low-glycemic load (this is explained in Chapter 7) – and by supplementing chromium.

Hormone imbalances, the most common being an underactive thyroid. The amino acid tyrosine, plus certain minerals, can make all the difference.

Food allergies and digestive problems. I will explain how your gut and your brain function are intimately connected.

Essential-fat deficiencies. Few of us get enough omega-3 fats, but these are the keys to healthy mood and brain function.

Neurotransmitter deficiencies. These are the key chemicals in the brain that affect mood. Some, such as serotonin, are made directly from amino acids, which are essential nutrients in your food. These amino acids can also be supplemented so that the deficiencies can be rapidly corrected. Finding out which amino acids will most help you can make all the difference to how you feel.

Lack of sleep. This has a big effect on how you feel. Finding out how to sleep through the night so that you can wake up refreshed can be a missing piece in feeling a whole lot better.

B-vitamin deficiencies. Each one of us is different and some of us need ten times more of certain B vitamins than others. I'm going to show you how to find out if you are one of those people and how to boost your mood and concentration by achieving your optimum intake of B vitamins.

Sunlight and exercise. Very few people in the northern hemisphere achieve enough sunlight for their body to make vitamin D (which is made in the skin directly from sun exposure), or eat sufficient vitamin D in their diet, and this is now known to be a critical factor in boosting mood. Combining exercise – a mood booster in its own right – with being outdoors, is a great way to feel better. I'll also be explaining about vitamin D-rich foods and supplements, and the signs that indicate you might need them.

For each of these mood-boosting secrets you'll be able to find out which factor is most likely to apply to you, and exactly what you need to do to correct the imbalances. First, let's explore the non-nutritional factors that affect how you feel.

Chapter 2

ARE YOU LETTING THOUGHTS AND FEELINGS SABOTAGE YOUR HAPPINESS?

Happiness is an elusive thing. One minute you have it, the next minute you don't. It is possible to feel happy even when things appear to be 'bad', and unhappy when everything seems to be OK. Has that ever happened to you? Of course, how you feel isn't simply a function of your chemistry or what you have been eating. In this chapter I'd like to delve into the psychological factors that have a big impact on how you feel. So, what is it that makes you feel good one minute and down the next? Is it purely a result of what's happening in your life? Let's explore this.

First, try this simple exercise.

EXERCISE: VISUALISING

1 Bring to mind, right now, a time when you were blissfully happy. Maybe you'd fallen in love, just got the best job or were lying on the beach on holiday. Scroll through the times you have been really happy, then pick one.

2 Now focus on one moment. Close your eyes and picture yourself in that moment. Imagine what you are wearing, who is there, what's around you. Now recall and relive the feeling of happiness until you are actually experiencing it; revel in the feeling.

3 Now keep the feeling, but let go of the circumstances. Stay with the feeling as you open your eyes and return to your current set of circumstances.

You may need to repeat the exercise to feel the experience of it fully, but it illustrates how happiness is not conditional on anything as such. Having said that, it is certainly true that particular conditions will help; for example, if you are lonely, finding the right man or woman may help; if you are broke, getting some money is most welcome; if you are out of work, getting a job makes you feel much better. But a kind word, or an unkind word, can make such a difference to our state of mind at any given moment.

We all have needs – for security, to be loved, a sense of self-esteem and so on – and having your needs fulfilled does help. We also have biological needs, such as the need for an even blood sugar level, hormonal balance, and enough vitamins, minerals and essential fats. We'll be delving into these needs in the chapters that follow.

How you feel in any given moment is an interplay between your state of mind, your circumstances and your biology, but let's keep exploring your state of mind, because to understand what makes you feel low, you need to also understand how experiences from your past resurface to affect the present and create a block to finding happiness.

Negative self-talk perpetuates our feelings of sadness

Our emotional state comes from the words and thoughts we have. Someone says something to us, or gives us a disapproving look, and we have a thought such as, *I'm not good enough/I'm unattractive/I'm a failure/I'll never...* or any one of hundreds of negative feelings we have about ourselves. This is called 'negative self-talk'. To make this more real for you, think of at least five repetitive thoughts you have that would fit into the category of negative self-talk, and write them down right now. (You'll find a list of the most commonly reported ones on page 170.)

These kinds of thoughts, or internal framings, are like deep grooves in our psyche and often stem from core early experiences, usually implanted from interactions with our parents. They shape us so strongly that we actually attract situations again and again that reinforce the exact same thoughts – and with those thoughts come all the horrible feelings of inadequacy, feeling useless, hopeless, damaged, unlovable, pathetic, inferior, unworthy, and so on. These kinds of feelings literally hijack our lives, creating physical pain as well as increased adrenal hormones (adrenalin and cortisol) and reduced serotonin which, in turn, make you more moody and irritable – as well as a host of other associated problems. It's a two-way street: feelings change your body's chemistry and your body's chemistry changes your feelings.

Healing the past

In Chapter 16 I'm going to show you how to identify these negative patterns and loosen the grip they hold on you. The first step to happiness is to build a good relationship with yourself and to heal relationships from the past. So often, when we identify the deep, negative thought patterns we have inherited, it brings us back to how our parents made us feel about ourselves. With that awareness often comes resentment. In Tim Laurence's excellent book *You Can Change Your Life*, there is the saying, 'we are all guilty, but not to blame'. The meaning here is that, for sure, your parents are guilty of helping you to build up your own library of negative thought patterns, as their parents were before them and, no doubt, you'll pass them on to your own children. These patterns are almost like our psychological 'genes' that get passed on from generation to generation. That's the way it works. But you can break free in the sense of firstly becoming aware of these negative thought patterns, and then putting some distance between them and who you really are.

Clean your karma

As well as your inherited plethora of negative thought patterns, there are also circumstances in your life: those negative experiences that leave emotional scars until we no longer have the flexibility in our psyche to see the wonder in life. These experiences 'feed' negative thought patterns that literally make us bound to states of sadness, anger or fear. In the Hindu tradition these are called 'karmic' experiences.

KARMIC EXPERIENCES

A karmic experience is anything that happens which generates a negative emotion; for example, someone insults you. Now, the memory of that person saying those words, *and* the 'unworthy' feeling that goes with them, become stored in your psyche.

If you continue to receive these karmic experiences, you soon develop a pattern that is like a groove you become stuck in, which says, *I am unworthy*, or words to that effect (such as *I am unlovable/incompetent/a loser/a failure*). Of course, if your parents have already instilled that sense of incompleteness within you, all these experiences feed the idea that you are, in some way, not good enough. As a consequence, we spend our lives trying to be good enough: saying the right things, doing the right things, trying to be smart, looking good, hanging out with the right people – anything to create the impression that we are 'good enough'. Who are *you* trying to impress?

Part of the secret to feeling good is learning how to discharge the negative emotions and our accumulation of sadness, anger and fear. This is how you can clean your karma. (I'll go into this in more detail in Chapter 16.) These are massive drains on our energy and are the enemies of feeling good. All of these get in the way of our ability to experience the wonder of life and to approach each moment and each day with spontaneity.

One of the main purposes of psychotherapy is to give you insight into these inherited negative perceptions and to provide techniques that you can learn from to help you move on from the past. There are many different kinds of psychotherapy, which I'll explain in Chapter 16, but, broadly speaking, there's plenty of evidence that psychotherapy is highly effective in improving mood.[6]

Being present

Feelings are there to show you something. The trouble is we get caught up in them and think they are permanent fixtures. Feelings, such as being angry, sad or frustrated, are a part of what makes us thinking human beings. However, although we recognise they exist, we do not have to feel the victim of those feelings or that they control us.

We need to be fully present in each moment, without preoccupations, negative thoughts or judgements. As one saying tells us: 'The past is history, the future a mystery – all that exists is the present – it is a gift. That's why it is called the present.' This whole subject of being in the present is core to many techniques that lift you out of depression, or at least give you a perspective on what you are feeling.

Eckhart Tolle's book *The Power of Now* really does give you the experience of being present and is well worth reading. We often get caught up in our thoughts and feelings, thinking that there is something we must do to feel better. But so often there is nothing that needs to be done. Firstly, feelings do change, if you let yourself feel them. Resistance is persistence. Often the real reasons for feeling upset are not the ones your mind thinks of at the time. Truly being present with, and honest about, your feelings will show you the root of them more effectively than trying to think your way out of them, or justifying why you feel the way you do by blaming something or someone else.

Of course, it is hard to be present if you have a head full of negative self-talk and disgruntled feelings about yourself and the world around you. So, the first step is to clean up your house, so to speak, to learn how to become aware of, and then discharge, the charged experiences and negative patterns that you inevitably accumulate.

Using mindfulness to stay in the present

When you dwell over things that have happened in the past, they take up your mind space and drag you down. So, instead, practise being in the here and now, allowing yourself to get on with your life even if your mind is chattering about the things that trouble you. One way to train your mind to clear itself of endless chatter is by practising meditation: you still your mind and when thoughts arise, as they inevitably will, you simply label them as 'thought' and let them drift by. This quiet time can free your mind beyond the few minutes that you are actually sitting there meditating. I'll be talking about this in Chapter 16 and giving you plenty of evidence to show that developing the art of mindfulness has a major impact on how you feel.

There's nothing wrong with thoughts as such, but the purpose of mindfulness is to develop the art of being in the present beyond thoughts or feelings. Often, feelings persist precisely because we resist them.

Your feelings also have a physical connection. Next time you are feeling miserable or angry or frustrated, or whatever word you use to describe your current state, become aware instead of where in your body you are experiencing this feeling. Identify the actual place and the physical feeling. For example, you might be feeling a tightness in your solar plexus or an ache in your heart or chest. Allow yourself to feel it. Stay with this feeling, however uncomfortable it may be. It too will pass. That's the nature of thoughts and feelings. They arise and they subside.

Find yourself

Behind all thought and feelings is that which never changes: the deepest experience of 'I am', of awareness, of presence, or simply being, with no sense of lack or needing anything. It is so often this sense of our true 'self' that we lose in periods of depression. Of the top scorers in our 100% Health Survey, almost half reported having a 'peak' experience – essentially an opening of the heart, an experience of unity or an awareness of pure being beyond thought. This kind of experience and awareness is the goal of all mystical and spiritual practices, the purpose of which is to connect us with a profound experience of being that is beyond any sense of time or space that connects our internal world with the external world. We become the witness of both the dramas in the world around us and our own internal dramas created by our endless thoughts and feelings.

In my view, society's denial of the spiritual nature of who we are is fuelling depression, and I have found that people with a sense of spiritual connection, or a belief in some form of higher or greater consciousness, are happier and have a richer purpose in life.

As a psychologist who has studied the brain, it is obvious to me that the world is not as we see it. What we see, or experience through our eyes, ears and other senses is, in its rawest sense, energy. Our senses translate the different manifestations of this energy into colours, sounds, smells and so forth. From these we develop constructs such as 'table' and build up a language of concepts that become our shared experience of the world. From this language we build up an idea of who we are in relation to the world we perceive. The experience of everything as energy is what fired Einstein, but it is also what's behind every true spiritual path. It is the words of those who have touched or have access to this level of experience that inspire us. William Blake said, 'If the doors of perception were cleansed everything would appear to man as it is, infinite.'

In my 100% Health Survey I asked the healthiest people if they had ever had such an experience: 50 per cent had, 28 per cent weren't quite sure, and 22 per cent hadn't. So, this kind of experience is really quite common, and presumably available to all. (Of course, if you've really bought into your negative self-talk you may believe that you are incapable of such experiences.)

Find your deepest meaning

Sometimes, the lack of this experience, or where we miss the experience of our core being, our sense of self or soul, is what makes us feel depressed. We lose our sense of meaning or purpose in life. Perhaps, when the person we love dies, or betrays or leaves us, or if we lose our job or status in the world, we feel life is meaningless and that there is no higher intelligence or purpose as such. We lose our faith that all life's lessons give us an opportunity to learn and to grow. 'The unfolding of my life is not an issue of competence or control. It is an issue of faith,' says Anne Wilson-Shaef, author of *Living in Process*. This excellent book helps put you back in touch with your life's journey and purpose.

Life can be seen as an unfolding journey that gives us opportunities to learn and grow. When we lose any sense of life's purpose we lose our love of life. What we describe as 'love' is really some kind of experience of connection, and it can be with people, animals or nature, but we can also 'love' food, money, movies, sex, drugs or rock and roll. The danger, of course, is that we can become attached to that sense of pleasure –

perhaps the taste of our favourite chocolate dessert or the hit we feel when we take a drug – and become addicted in our desire to keep having more and more until the magic has gone from the experience.

Some of these experiences are just about sense pleasures, which, as you'll see, also have their roots in changes in brain chemistry, as does their desensitisation with overuse. This is the basis for addiction. In the next chapters I'll be explaining how specific nutrients and drugs both target the very same changes in brain chemistry that make us feel better.

Getting connected

There is another kind of love that doesn't increase the levels of 'feel-good' chemicals in your brain as such; one that is about the sense of connection, of unity. I remember one man who said, 'When I do good, I feel good. When I do bad, I feel bad. That is my religion.' Many people have an inner experience or belief in humanity as such and derive meaning from serving humanity or serving their community or family. Having such a sense of purpose or outlook on life not only improves your mood but it's positively good for your health; for example, having a sense of purpose in life is associated with halving the risk of Alzheimer's disease.[7] A scientist may be enthusiastic about using the tools of science to unravel the secrets of the world; an artist may be enthusiastic in the process of expressing his or her perception. Of course, we are all both scientists and artists in the process of understanding our world and expressing that meaning.

Enthusiasm and inspiration are certain attributes of the Feel Good Factor. Given that our world as we perceive it is made out of words, these particular words are also interesting. Enthusiasm literally means 'the god inside'. Inspire means 'to heighten, to exalt, to breathe in, to animate'. In a sense, these words describe that experience of being in a larger awareness that is in itself energising. We'll be exploring this more in Part 2 with practical ways that can help you rekindle your enthusiasm for life. Often, the first step is to re-energise yourself by correcting biochemical imbalances with optimum nutrition. However, if you do feel you've lost track, it is really important to find someone you can talk to, perhaps a close friend, a counsellor or a spiritual advisor. In the next chapter we'll explore non-psychological factors that affect how you feel.

Chapter 3

FEELING SAD IS NOT ALL IN THE MIND

How you feel day to day isn't purely a function of what's going on in your life and how you deal with it psychologically. You cannot have a single thought, or experience a feeling, without a corresponding change in your body's chemistry, and you cannot eat or drink anything without it having an effect on the sensitive chemistry in your brain. Outside factors, such as our exposure to the sun, the weather, and even the phases of the moon, have all been shown to have profound effects on how we feel. So too do physical activities such as exercise. Sex is especially effective, because it is a three-in-one package, causing a massive release of neurotransmitters – the brain's feel-good chemicals – as well as providing physical intimacy, plus physical exertion.

The very fact that a drink or a drug – whether it's Ecstasy or Prozac – can affect how you feel, is a clear illustration that anything that changes your brain's chemistry has the power to alter your mood and perception of the world. Sometimes we get hooked on these substances or behaviours that make us feel good. This can be the starting point for addiction if we need more and more of the same thing to feel good.

In this book, I'm going to show you how to create the best set of circumstances, through simple changes to your lifestyle, your diet and the use of specific supplements, to programme your body's chemistry for feeling good.

Can you change your genes?

You may ask, isn't our health, and even the tendency to experience low moods, just genetic or inherited? If there are other members of your family who have a tendency towards feeling low, or who have suffered from depression, I'm sure you've wondered whether it's 'in the genes', maybe fearing that there's nothing you can do about it. If so, you are both right and wrong.

There are genes that you can inherit that make you more prone to feeling low. One of these is a sequence called 'reward deficiency' genes. If you inherit these genes, it's harder to feel satisfied. People who have them – about one person in ten – also have fewer receptors for dopamine, a major feel-good chemical in the brain. As a consequence, they are more likely to gravitate towards substances and behaviours that give them a kick-start. This can include taking risks, seeking endless adventures, falling in love, drinking or taking drugs. Many become addicted to searching for something that makes them feel satisfied.

You can be in control

Although the genes you inherit are there for life, whether or not a gene is activated or 'expressed' depends on factors you *can* control, including diet and social aspects; for example, we know that animals deprived of maternal care become prone to reacting badly to stress (as seen in research on baby rats that were deprived of licking and grooming by the mother in early infancy).[8] In adulthood, if they are given nutrients that are required for switching genes on or off, this switches off the over-reaction.[9] Other research, which was carried out on 500 people, tested for five potentially negative gene mutations that meant certain enzymes in the body become less efficient at doing their job. The researchers found that about one person in ten had one or more of these gene mutations. They then gave the volunteers B vitamins and found that, in four out of five, the supplement could restore the defective enzymes to normal function.[10]

This might sound too good to be true, but I've seen people who are drowning in suicidal and irrational thoughts literally restored to a stable state of mind just by taking specific B vitamins. There are even double-blind controlled trials showing that the right B vitamins in the correct amounts can give substantial relief to people with mental-health problems. I'll be talking about these in Chapter 13, because taking B vitamins is one of my top ten mood-boosting secrets.

Your mind and body are not separate

One of the inherent problems in our cultural thinking about mood is the separation of mind and body. The philosopher René Descartes did us a great disservice by promoting the notion of a separation between our mind (the thinking thing) and our body – the former being the domain of psychotherapists and the latter the domain of your doctor. Few psychotherapists learn about brain chemistry and the impact of nutrients on mood, while few scientists have knowledge of the 'soft' sciences of understanding the nature of the mind. The true science of feeling good involves both changing how you relate to the world you experience and to changing that world – in other words, changing your environment. The environment I am describing here isn't just the environment outside your body but also the environment inside your body, and the biggest factor that affects this is what you eat and drink.

In fact, it's hard to separate your 'inner' and 'outer' environment; for example, exposing your skin to sunlight makes you feel good, because it actually raises serotonin (the mood-boosting neurotransmitter) levels in the brain. One of the ways it does this is by converting cholesterol into vitamin D in the skin. But you can also eat vitamin D; rich sources are found in oily fish such as mackerel. Supplementing vitamin D also helps to improve your mood. In Chapter 14 I'm going to explain about upping your vitamin D level and some simple ways you can get a mood and energy boost using a 60 watt light bulb. In Chapter 14 I'll also explain what kind of exercise has the best mood-boosting effects.

Let there be light

We usually think of light as something external – from the sun. But is there an inner light?

Your brain is tuned into light. There is an ebb and flow of different chemicals during the cycle of day and night. At night the brain makes more melatonin. This, itself, is a natural antidepressant and sleep promoter. If you are jet-lagged and out of sync with the earth's day–night cycle, taking melatonin helps to bring you back into balance and give you a good night's sleep. Later on, in Chapter 14, I'll be explaining how to get more light, and more vitamin D – itself made from light – and how this can literally help to 'enlighten' you.

Sleep – are you getting enough?

A lack of sleep is a major factor in how you feel. We all need a good seven hours of uninterrupted sleep, but few of us get it. In our 100% Health Survey, 55 per cent of people said that they had difficulty sleeping or had restless sleep, while 63 per cent said they needed more sleep. One of the outcomes of following the Feel Good Factor programme is better quality sleep. Chapter 12 explains how to achieve this.

Every part of your body relies on the food you eat to make it work efficiently. Both melatonin and serotonin are made from tryptophan, a simple amino acid found in protein. The ability to turn tryptophan into serotonin, and then melatonin, depends on a whole host of nutrients, including those mood-boosting B vitamins, as well as the minerals zinc and magnesium, available from food but not always in sufficient quantities. I'll be recommending a diet that provides these kinds of nutrients as well as supplements for those vitamins and minerals your body is lacking.

Are you serotonin depleted?

Anything that affects serotonin levels tends to affect your mood – and some of us are deficient. Women, for example, are more likely to be deficient than men, especially under conditions of prolonged stress – which includes not getting enough sleep. Also, if your diet isn't up to scratch, you may not be getting an optimal intake of the key nutrients necessary to make enough. A lack of serotonin also leads to sugar cravings, whereas having enough will curb your appetite. That's one of the good side effects of the Feel Good Factor programme: your appetite becomes normal and you will stop craving sugar. If you have gained weight, you are likely to lose it.

If you are one of those people who craves something sweet when you are feeling down, and feels better after eating it, you may be low in serotonin. Whether you are or not, and what to do about it if you are, is the subject of Chapter 11.

Chemical ways that serotonin can be raised

One of the classic drugs that raises serotonin, albeit for a few hours, is MDMA (Ecstasy). When people take this drug, they often feel temporarily much happier and more connected. But if you give someone on Ecstasy a plate of the most delicious food, they won't be interested in eating a mouthful. Serotonin levels have a powerful effect on appetite as well as mood.

It is serotonin's mood-boosting effect that is exploited in antidepressant drugs, called SSRIs (or selective serotonin reuptake inhibitors). Why then are nutrients not prescribed instead of SSRIs? The answer is that although nutrients provide the raw materials to make things like neurotransmitters, they can't be patented and are therefore not profitable as medicines. SSRIs, however, work in a different way, by blocking the brain's ability to break down serotonin; but because they are man-made chemicals they are therefore patentable. The result is that the drugs, which are highly profitable to the companies who make them, are marketed as the answer to depression and widely prescribed, in spite of their high cost. SSRI drugs, such as Prozac, stop your brain breaking down serotonin once it has done its job, which is what the brain normally does. As a consequence, you have more serotonin and a better mood – at least, that's the idea. But how effective are these antidepressants and what about their side effects? I examine this in the next chapter.

Chapter 4

THE DOWNSIDE OF ANTIDEPRESSANTS

If you are feeling depressed or excessively anxious, or if you can't sleep, the chances are you'll visit your doctor. In fact, about a third of GP visits involve people presenting with these kinds of psychological issues. Many leave with a prescription for a drug, be it an antidepressant, a sleeping pill or some kind of tranquilliser. I am going to show you that antidepressants are less effective, and have many more undesirable side effects, than a nutritional approach.

The first obvious anomaly is that the diagnosis, for example of depression, is made purely on the basis of psychological symptoms and tests, such as the Ham-D scale explained on page 9. Yet the treatment given is chemical. That assumes that the 'cause' of depression is a biochemical imbalance – and one that can be corrected by drugs.

If you are prescribed an antidepressant, you will usually be told that you are low in serotonin and that these drugs boost it. The idea is that drugs such as Prozac and other SSRIs give you more serotonin in the brain by blocking the ability of the brain to break it down. At the Brain Bio Centre, however, we test serotonin levels (more on this later), but we have found that although some people are indeed deficient others are not.

> If you are taking antidepressants at the moment, or thinking about it, make sure you also pursue the nutritional approach. Should you decide, with your doctor's support, to come off medication, the nutritional approach also helps minimise withdrawal effects.

The happy pills

SSRIs largely replaced the former most popular antidepressants in the 1990s, called tricyclic antidepressants (such as amitriptyline), with claims that they would bring instant happiness and even the suggestion that we could all benefit from taking them. Prozac (fluoxetine) led the way. The name suggested you could be pro-active: a professional with extra zappiness. It was happiness in a pill, not just for those who were depressed, but for all of us, and it offered the promise of instant bliss. It was almost hip to be on Prozac, and any suggestion of side effects was downplayed.

Most SSRIs are now off-patent and are being replaced by the new generation of antidepressants called SNRIs (serotonin and noradrenalin reuptake inhibitors). These drugs are based on the revised position that depressed people can also be deficient in another neurotransmitter called noradrenalin, the cousin of adrenalin, which leads to a lack of drive and motivation. But do any doctors test for noradrenalin deficiency before prescribing these drugs? The answer is no, but it is something we do at the Brain Bio Centre where we find, as before, that although some people are deficient others are not. These SNRI drugs, and others like them, are the new money-makers of the pharmaceutical industry now that SSRIs are off-patent.

The profit in antidepressants

Antidepressants are big business. In 2004 four brands of antidepressants made $10 billion in sales, while three brands of anti-psychotic medication made $9.4 billion. By 2005, 27 million Americans – that's one person in ten – had been prescribed antidepressants. And today, who knows how many people are on medication? What's more, among antidepressant users, the number of those who were also prescribed anti-psychotic drugs – originally developed for psychotic conditions such as schizophrenia – was about one person in ten, compared to one in five who were offered psychotherapy.[11] In both the US and the UK there has been a massive increase in doctors diagnosing bipolar disorder, leading them to prescribe both an antidepressant and an anti-psychotic drug. Anti-psychotic drugs (such as Zyprexa) are now among the top-ten selling drugs.

By 2008, sales of antidepressants in the US alone were worth almost $10 billion with 164 million prescriptions written annually and global sales estimated at about twice this amount.[12] In 2009 global sales of Cymbalta (duloxetine), one of the new generation antidepressants, exceeded $3 billion, overtaking its closest rival Effexor, which will soon be off-patent. The makers, Wyeth, are now moving their marketing muscle behind a new, but similar kind of, drug called Pristiq. Together, antidepressant and anti-psychotic drugs are bringing in over $30 billion a year for the pharmaceutical industry. But do they work?

Seeing through the fairytale

It's a fairly consistent theme in the history of drugs that the new patented and profitable generation of drugs are claimed to be better than those they replace. That was certainly the case with the Prozac generation of SSRIs. As long ago as 2000, a large study, based on all the best evidence submitted to the US Food and Drug Administration over ten years for SSRI licence applications, concluded that these drugs were actually no better than the older 'tricyclic' antidepressants (such as amitriptyline).[13]

We are also often led to believe that these mass-prescribed drugs are well researched and well proven, but psychology professor Dr Irving Kirsch, author of a book called *The Emperor's New Drugs*, believes that much of the apparent benefit of these drugs is a sham.

Kirsch's analysis, which has been published in leading medical journals such as the *British Medical Journal*,[14] shows that much of the apparent benefit of these drugs is due to an 'enhanced placebo effect'. He shows that, firstly, most people on these trials guess that they are on antidepressants because of the side effects. When you sign up for these trials you are given a long list of potential side effects from nausea to sleeping problems that you may experience if you are assigned to the drug group, not the placebo group. As a result, many people soon guess which group they are in. Kirsch has shown that if a person experiences side effects, they tend to rate their improvement as better, thinking that they are on the real thing. The small difference between antidepressant response and placebo is simply explained by an enhanced placebo response. In trials where placebos that also induce side effects are given, there's no difference! There's also no evidence that increasing the dose works, which is what most doctors do (although, with more side effects there may be a further enhanced placebo effect). Also, most reported benefit occurs in the first two weeks, so the often-used explanation that you just haven't taken them for long enough is again not true.

How we are led to believe these drugs are the answer

These drug trials are really important because, without a positive result, a drug company can't get a licence to market the drug, which is a signal to doctors and patients that the drugs are safe and, more importantly, effective. What is perhaps rather crazy is that, until recently, a drug company could run dozens of trials, of which many may have proved the drug to be ineffective, but only submit those that showed a 'positive' effect, to acquire the licence. This loophole is now being tightened up, thanks to the work of people like Kirsch, by requiring that any proposed trial must enter a register and can only be published if it has done so. In this way negative results can't be so easily hidden. But, as Kirsch points out, as long as the regulator (the MHRA in Britain and the FDA in America) is paid for by the pharmaceutical industry, we are unlikely to see fair play.

Natural remedies are sidelined

The law states that any treatment that claims to treat, prevent or cure a disease (such as depression) must have a medical licence. But the cost of a medical licence is so prohibitive that it is rarely granted to any treatment that doesn't have a patent, meaning the treatment is man-made and capable of being monopolised, giving a potentially highly profitable return. Many of the extremely effective nutrients I'll be recommending later in the book – ranging from B vitamins, chromium, essential fats and amino acids – can't be patented because they already exist in nature. Therefore, even if they work, supplement companies have to keep quiet, otherwise their product will be classified as a medicine, and it then becomes illegal. This is exactly what happened to one highly effective amino acid, SAMe (more on this later), which is now no longer available in Europe. Of course, man-made drugs are far more likely to induce side effects than nutrients that have been around for millennia. The fact is, we have a legal framework that makes governments and pharmaceutical companies rich, but it fails to deliver safe and effective medicine to the people.

How effective are antidepressants?

Politics and placebo effects aside, just how effective are antidepressants? A meta-analysis of six large studies published in the *Journal of the American Medical Association* found that for people with moderate depression (with a Ham-D score below 23), which accounts for the vast majority of people with diagnosed depression, antidepressants are really no better than a placebo.[15] To quote the study: 'The magnitude of benefit of antidepressant medication compared with placebo increases with severity of depression symptoms and may be minimal or nonexistent, on average, in patients with mild or moderate symptoms. For patients with very severe depression, the benefit of medications over placebo is substantial.'

A recent report on all treatments for depression from the UK's National Institute for Health and Clinical Excellence (NICE) agrees: 'There is little clinically important difference between antidepressants and placebo for mild depression.'[16] For mild depression, NICE does not recommend antidepressants, favouring instead exercise, 'guided self-help' (such as keeping a journal) and counselling. Unfortunately, nutrition has not yet made it on to their agenda. But just how substantial is the benefit even for those with severe depression?

A slight improvement over placebos

Most trials show that placebos give a 50 per cent improvement in the Ham-D scale whereas most antidepressants give a 65 per cent improvement. So that's a 15 per cent improvement. What does this actually mean? If you had ticked three fewer questions in the mood check on page 7 that would be the equivalent of a 15 per cent improvement – the average achieved for antidepressant medication. This is a tiny difference and one that Kirsch believes is explained by the enhanced placebo effect. While not everyone agrees with Kirsch's analysis, there is little doubt that the benefits of antidepressants have been vastly exaggerated. The publication *Newsweek* produced an insightful report into antidepressants entitled 'The Depressing News about Antidepressants' (available online at www.newsweek.com/id/232781/page/1, if you'd like to know more about the evidence and the controversies). So that's the scale of the potential benefits. What about the side effects?

The side effects are depressing

What's really worrying about antidepressant drugs are their side effects, which include at least a doubling of the risk of suicide, sexual dysfunction, insomnia, nausea, diarrhoea, sweating and drowsiness, a possible increased risk of heart disease and, recently, some concerns about negative effects on babies in pregnant women taking antidepressants. All in all, they're a bad deal.

Tricyclic antidepressants such as amitriptyline, Anafranil and Prothiadin have over 20 side effects listed in the doctor's drug guide, the *British National Formulary*, including dry mouth, blurred vision, nausea, confusion, cardiovascular problems, sweating, tremors and behavioural disturbance.[17] Monoamine oxidase inhibitors (MAOIs) such as Nardil and Parstelin have even worse side effects, and can be very difficult to stop taking, as they're highly addictive. They can cause dangerously high blood pressure if taken with substances containing yeast, alcohol or caffeine. Some patients have died after taking MAOIs having failed to avoid these substances, which are found hidden in many convenience foods.

SSRIs were originally touted as having fewer side effects for most people, but they can create profound problems in a significant minority. Prozac, the market leader, prescribed to more than 38 million people worldwide, has 45 side effects listed in the *British National Formulary*. According to psychiatrist David Richman, between 10 and 25 per cent of people experience each of the following: nausea, nervousness, insomnia, headache, tremors, anxiety, drowsiness, dry mouth, excessive sweating and diarrhoea. These drugs also tend to flatten moods, sometimes to the point of zombie-like emotionlessness, or cause people to feel fuzzy. SSRIs can also trigger major sexual dysfunction, resulting in an inability to climax in both men and women (in its turn leading to a loss of intimacy that, ironically, could adversely affect a person's ability to come out of depression).

On top of this, research published in 2006 suggests that SSRIs might dramatically increase the risk of death in people with cardiovascular disease.[18] There have now been 90 legal actions and one successful litigation, with $6.4 million being awarded against Eli Lilly, the makers of Prozac.

Antidepressants increase the risk of suicide

As I explained in the Introduction, Prozac and another commonly prescribed antidepressant, Seroxat, have shown clear evidence of agitation leading to potential aggressive and suicidal behaviour in as many as a quarter of patients in a number of clinical trials; however, these particular SSRI antidepressants shouldn't be singled out. Most antidepressants increase suicidal tendencies. A review of 702 studies on SSRI antidepressants showed that people taking an SSRI were more than twice as likely to attempt suicide compared with those taking a dummy pill. The researchers also noted that the actual number of suicide attempts is likely to be much higher, because many of the studies did not gather this information.[19] 'I estimate that about one person a day has committed suicide as a direct result of taking Prozac since it was introduced,' says one of the authors, Dr David Healy, who first petitioned the UK government's Medicine Control Agency to warn users about the potential adverse reactions some 15 years ago.[20]

The first study to show a link between an SSRI and suicide was published in 1990.[21] Between 1995 and 2002, Dr David Healy, who was worried about the link between SSRIs and suicide, sent hundreds of pages of evidence about it to the UK Medicines and Healthcare Products Regulatory Agency. The MHRA continued to insist there was no problem.[22] In 2000, a patent for a new sort of Prozac was found to have been filed by the manufacturers of the original version. It claimed that the new version did not cause the suicidal thoughts the way the old version had.[23]

In 2004, 3.5 million people received 20 million prescriptions for SSRIs,[24] and global sales of SSRIs were about $17 billion.[25] Then government agencies started to go public with concerns about safety, but by then the patents were running out in any case. Healy's book, *Let Them Eat Prozac*, exposes the extraordinary resistance the pharmaceutical industry and government agencies (who are partly paid for by the industry) have shown in acknowledging the dangers of antidepressants.

The new SNRI antidepressants are no better

A fourth generation of antidepressants is largely replacing the SSRIs as their patents run out. These SNRIs come with side effects too: nausea, headaches, insomnia, sleepiness, dry mouth, dizziness, constipation, weakness, sweating, nervousness and, as with SSRIs, serious sexual dysfunction. Do they also increase the risk of suicide? During trials of Cymbalta, before it was licensed in 2004, there was at least one 'unexplained' suicide by a 19-year-old girl. In 2005, the FDA warned that a 'higher than expected rate of suicide attempts was observed' among patients taking it.[26] But how long will it take before government agencies take note and publicise warnings? For SSRIs it took ten years – just long enough for the patents to run out.

I have seen no evidence that makes me believe the newer antidepressants are going to prove any safer. Furthermore, in our clinical experience at the Brain Bio Centre, they are often even harder to give up.

CASE STUDY: FRAN

Fran was feeling extremely low after a bereavement and went to see her doctor, who prescribed antidepressants and referred her for counselling, In her words:

'I assumed that was what you did when you felt low. Two years later I had gained 6 stone [84lb/38kg], had severe memory loss and just about every muscle in my body was cramped. Whenever I tried to explain these concerns to my doctor it was like I was speaking a different language. I couldn't get out of bed, my legs would buckle and then I'd collapse. Self-confidence was absolutely nil and I tried lots of different things, including reading the medical literature. I realised that there wasn't a lot of consensus on what actually causes depression. I read every self-help book going, changed my diet, got colonics, spiritual healing – you name it, I tried it! But I just seemed to be getting worse. I even tried to wean myself off the drugs twice, but that made things worse. I felt that I was between a rock and a hard place.'

Eventually, someone gave Fran one of my earlier books:

'I read Optimum Nutrition for the Mind, cover to cover that night, and it was so exciting after all those years of feeling completely loopy every time I tried to ask for help to realise that there might really be something out there. I asked my GP – because at this stage my brain was so fried, and for all I knew these guys could be charlatans. I gave him the book and said, "Look, would you mind just having a quick read and telling me is this for real? Would this be viable?" And he did, and he told me to go for it. Interestingly enough, when I told the psychiatrist, I was threatened with hospitalisation, so I decided to trust my GP on that one. I made an appointment with the Brain Bio Centre. It was just so exciting to be asked sensible questions and to be treated like an intelligent person. When the tests came back, it was beyond empowering. To have Lorraine actually say to me, "I'm looking at these results and I'm wondering how on earth you've even gotten out of bed!" She wasn't calling me lazy or a negative thinker. So we designed a supplement plan, and in one month I started noticing changes. By April of this year [five months later], I had made such progress that I was actually investigated for benefit fraud. The only way to clear my name was to show receipts of supplements and the treatments.

'By June, I completed the coast-to-coast walk – all 200 miles of it – carrying my own gear. By July, I sat a ten-day meditation course and by August I was working full-time *and going to the gym every day. Just last week, Lorraine and I designed my maintenance plan so that from now on I can manage my treatment myself. I just wanted to thank you very much.'*

Are antidepressants addictive?

Ten years ago, research alluded to the 'cessation effects' of many antidepressants. Authorities, such as the MHRA in the UK and the FDA in the US, demanded that drug companies come clean and refer to 'withdrawal effects' instead.

Of course, all of this is semantics, and there's a thin line between 'withdrawal effects' and addiction. What you and I mean by addictive is: if you stop the substance you feel lousy, and you crave it to relieve your suffering. That's exactly what happens to many people who try to stop taking antidepressants. Although SSRI antidepressants may not be technically addictive, there is now considerable evidence that the majority of those who try to quit experience alarming withdrawal symptoms. One study testing withdrawal showed that as many as 85 per cent of the volunteers – people with no previous hint of depression – suffered with agitation, abnormal dreams, insomnia and other adverse effects.[27] In studies on Cymbalta 44 per cent of people reported adverse symptoms on discontinuation, compared to 22 per cent on placebo.[28] A Canadian study also found about a quarter of people had withdrawal symptoms on stopping SSRIs.[29]

CASE STUDY: CHRISTIANNE

> At the age of 18, Christianne was prescribed Prozac and then Seroxat for her depression and panic attacks. Here's what happened when she started taking the drug, and then when she tried to stop:
>
> *'Since being on Seroxat I've started self-harming – cutting myself – and I also have a disturbed sleep pattern. When I do sleep, I have very vivid, weird dreams and violent nightmares and I sweat excessively. I have feelings of inadequacy and suicidal thoughts on a daily basis, and I hate myself for it. I've often wanted to overdose on my*

sleeping tablets so I wouldn't have to wake up in the morning, and I have sometimes taken two instead of one before going to bed. I feel more withdrawn than before, I have difficulty getting up in the mornings and I have violent mood swings, which is quite out of character for me. I suffer from extreme headaches and spells of light-headedness, which sometimes makes me lose my balance. I also become confused quickly and have spells of feeling "spaced-out" with an awful concentration span. I get upset and emotional very quickly, sometimes for the silliest of reasons. Sometimes I have no appetite at all.

'I feel worse now than I ever did before. I mentioned these feelings to my doctor at the mental health clinic and she told me that these feelings weren't side effects from the drug, but totally psychological and that they were down to the development of my condition, which I do not believe to be the case. When I asked her what she was going to do about the way I was feeling, she said she would refer me to a psychologist. Six months later, I am still waiting for an appointment to come through. She also suggested upping the dosage to 40mg, which I refused.

'My last spell of self-harm led to an argument between my long-term boyfriend and me. It was after this that I decided to come off my tablets completely, as my thought was that I couldn't feel much worse than I do now; however, no more than a day or two after, I began suffering severe withdrawal symptoms. These included an extreme feeling of weakness, excessive and painful diarrhoea, stomach cramps, intense nausea and the shakes. I felt so ill that I began taking the tablets again that evening and I am still taking them today.

'I am still on these tablets and want to come off them. I wonder if I will ever feel "normal" again. These tablets have ruined my life. I believe that it is these tablets that make me feel and behave the way I do. I feel enormously angry with the doctors and medical associations for dismissing these symptoms out of hand.'

However, Christianne attended the Brain Bio Centre where she was treated with the nutritional approach described in this book. It has been so effective that she no longer needs antidepressants and no longer suffers from depression or panic attacks.

Given that both antidepressants and anti-psychotic medication appear to be addictive for some, in the sense that the terrible withdrawal effects such as those experienced by Christianne motivate their continuation, one has to question whether modern psychiatry has made a Faustian bargain, swapping a rather small short-term improvement for long-term drug dependency at a scale never before seen.

Coming off antidepressants

In my opinion, antidepressants should be used only as a last resort, and even then, only for a short period of time, especially since equally effective but much safer alternatives exist, as you will discover in Part 2.

If you are currently on antidepressants and would like to come off them, the best strategy is to phase out the antidepressant and phase in the nutrients and herbs I describe, which help to promote a good mood but without the side effects. You should definitely do this only with the support of your doctor, and preferably with the guidance of a nutritional therapist (see Resources). With the correct nutritional support it is much easier.

DIRTY MEDICINE

Advocates of pharmaceutical medicine often argue that the only good science is large-scale placebo-controlled trials. The *British Medical Journal*[30] published a good article about the dangers of medicine only taking into account placebo-controlled trial results. The trouble with these trials is that they only really work for testing pills, thus playing into the hands of the pharmaceutical industry. They also cost, on average, about £5 million each. Lifestyle factors, such as exercise and nutrition, aren't amenable to this kind of research and, anyway, there's not that kind of money floating around for non-patentable treatments. Of course there's the enhanced placebo effect, mentioned earlier, which makes a mockery of most drug trials, since most drugs do have noticeable side effects, hence it isn't hard for a volunteer to guess that they are on a drug and not a placebo.

CONTINUED...

Unfortunately, it gets worse. You might have wondered whether any of these trial results gets fudged. After all, there's big money at stake. A recent review set out to explore this.[31] In surveys that asked about the behaviour of research colleagues, 14 per cent knew someone who had fabricated, falsified or altered data, and up to 72 per cent knew someone who had committed other questionable research practices. Misconduct was reported most frequently by medical and pharmacological researchers.

Furthermore, it's not just the science that gets distorted, it's also the marketing. In 2009 Pfizer got the biggest ever parking ticket, paying $2.3 billion to resolve federal criminal and civil charges that it had illegally promoted some of its drugs. This, together with the large-scale suppression of information about side effects, means we end up with a type of medicine that is largely dependent on drugs, and for drugs such as antidepressants, once you are on them it's often hard to come off. But, there is a better way.

Natural antidepressants work better

In the next chapter, and in Part 2, we are going to look at some of the most effective natural remedies that have helped people like Fran and Christianne get their lives back on track. We're going to examine the effects of certain nutrients such as folic acid, B_{12} and chromium, as well as essential omega-3 fats and amino acids such as 5-HTP. The results of placebo-controlled trials are more likely to be real, and not an enhanced placebo effect as is the case for antidepressant drugs. These nutrients have no noticeable side effects, so there would be no obvious way of knowing if you were taking part in a placebo-controlled trial, or guessing whether you were taking chromium or B vitamins, for example. The nutritional approaches, already proven in double-blind trials, are more likely to produce real results in a placebo-controlled trial rather than an enhanced placebo effect seen with side-effect causing drugs.

Finding the right combination of nutrients for you is often more effective than antidepressant drugs, and a lot safer. This book will help you do just that.

IMPORTANT NOTE IF YOU ARE ON ANTIDEPRESSANT MEDICATION

You can take almost all the nutrients described alongside medication, with the exception of 5-HTP (see page 42), making you feel better and helping to minimise side effects when you come off medication; however, don't come off medication without consulting your doctor. If you'd like help with minimising withdrawal effects, it is best to consult a qualified nutritional therapist or come to the Brain Bio Centre. At the Brain Bio Centre we have experienced psychiatrists who can help people withdraw from medication. Some of the recent anti-psychotic drugs given for depression are extremely dangerous to stop suddenly.

Chapter 5

NATURE'S PROVEN BLUES BUSTERS

If how you feel is partly caused by imbalances in the brain's sensitive chemistry, whether to do with psychological, diet or lifestyle factors, it makes more sense to rebalance it using chemicals that are part of our evolutionary design – that is, nutrients – rather than drugs. This was the thinking of the early pioneers of a whole new approach to medicine, called 'orthomolecular' medicine ('orthomolecular' means 'the right molecules'). Pioneers such as Dr Abram Hoffer, a psychiatrist from Canada caring for hundreds of schizophrenic patients, and twice Nobel Prize winner Dr Linus Pauling, discovered that when a person is sick their health can be restored by using the same nutrients necessary to maintain health, but in larger amounts.

Vitamin C is a classic example. Our jungle-dwelling ancestors would have consumed something like 1g (1,000mg) of vitamin C a day from fresh fruits, berries and vegetables. That's the equivalent of 22 supermarket oranges. Nowadays, we struggle to achieve 100mg; that's why many people supplement 1g a day, which is a good way to maintain healthy immunity as well as reducing your risk of many diseases. But if you have a cold, even this amount isn't enough. Taking 1g a day might slightly shorten the length of the cold and reduce the symptoms, but if you take 1g *an hour* at the onset of a cold, the symptoms will rarely last more than 12 hours. When you are ill, you will need more than the maintenance level to recover. In this book I will help you to discern which nutrients you are low in and I will then recommend higher doses than you'll need once you are feeling better, to redress those imbalances.

Why the larger amounts?

Dr Abram Hoffer, working in Saskatchewan back in the 1960s, found that those people with mental-health problems responded much better to large amounts of vitamin C and B vitamins. It is also entirely possible that those prone to depression or anxiety may genetically require greater levels of certain nutrients compared to other people. This has certainly been found in children with autism and adults with schizophrenia; for example, people with schizophrenia need to take in more vitamin C to achieve the same blood level as someone without the condition.[32]

Following the work of these pioneers, a whole host of nutrients have been discovered that are often deficient, but which can, in large amounts, bring your brain's sensitive chemistry back into balance and improve your mood considerably. These include:

- The amino acids tryptophan, 5-HTP and S-adenosyl methionine, known as SAMe
- The B vitamins, niacin (B_3) pyridoxine (B_6), folic acid and B_{12}
- Omega-3 fats, especially EPA
- Vitamin D
- The minerals zinc, magnesium and chromium
- The herb St John's wort

If your brain's chemistry is out of balance, getting the right combination of these is usually a lot more effective than simply taking an antidepressant drug.

The Brain Bio Centre approach

When clients come to the Brain Bio Centre we not only assess their mood using the Ham-D scale but we also take a sample of blood, urine and even hair to analyse imbalances in the body's chemistry. This includes measuring the neurotransmitter status, the level of essential nutrients such as vitamin D, essential fats, vitamins and minerals. We also screen for hormone imbalances and food allergies. From this we develop a personalised nutritional programme of diet and supplements, together with recommended lifestyle changes.

CASE STUDY: FRANK

Frank was 48 when he came to see us. He had suffered from depression, with occasional manic spells, all his life. He'd tried both Prozac and Seroxat, but they'd made him feel worse and occasionally suicidal. Counselling and homeopathy hadn't helped either. When he arrived at the Brain Bio Centre he scored 22 on the Ham-D scale, indicating major depression. Blood tests, among others, showed he had low serotonin and suboptimum levels of many minerals, as well as having some food allergies. He was given supplements, including essential fats, 5-HTP (a naturally occurring chemical the brain uses to make serotonin) and a vitamin B complex, as well as a diet that avoided his food allergens. He was also encouraged to exercise. Eight months later he reported feeling 'happy, healthy and fit' and his score on the Ham-D scale had dropped by 19 points. That's an 86 per cent drop. Remember how antidepressants generally lower the score by 15 per cent (see page 29)? An SSRI drug can be licensed if it lowers a Ham-D score by just three points!

CASE STUDY: HANNAH

Hannah had suffered from depression for seven years. She was overweight and suffered from poor digestion. She had tried antidepressants but did not feel comfortable taking them. When she first attended the Brain Bio Centre she felt socially withdrawn, had no motivation, was forgetful and confused and never felt refreshed from sleep.

Tests revealed she was deficient in magnesium, omega-3 fats and vitamin D, so Hannah was given a supplement programme and dietary advice to get optimally nourished. Within two months her mood, energy and digestion were greatly improved. By month three she described how she felt as 'dramatically different. My mood is great, it's easier to get up in the mornings and I have even joined a gym!'

Recognising the differences

These two cases illustrate a few key points if you want to recover your Feel Good Factor. The first is that we are not all the same. The idea that any one drug, herb or supplement, type of psychotherapy or lifestyle change is going to work for each one of us is naive. This is simply because we are complex beings, and how we feel is a result of complex influences, including our genetics, upbringing, life experiences, mind frame, nutrition and other environmental factors, including light and exercise.

If your car isn't working, the first thing a mechanic has to do is diagnose the problem. I find it extraordinary that, given all the advances in nutritional medicine, a person presenting with the symptoms of depression is rarely checked for neurotransmitter or nutritional deficiencies, or even something simple such as thyroid function – since having an underactive thyroid is another potential cause for feeling tired and low. In Part 2, I'm going to show you the main avenues you need to explore to restore your *joie de vivre*, how to test for potential imbalances, and then how to build your own mood-boosting programme.

The second point is that Frank's and Hannah's treatment involved a number of different nutrients. Although there are positive studies for each one, it is the combination of the correct cocktail of nutrients that gives you the quickest recovery. I'm going to show you how to find out what cocktail of nutrients is right for you to make a speedy recovery. Here's a quick run through of the kinds of factors and remedies we find most effective at the Brain Bio Centre.

Natural serotonin enhancers

I've already mentioned serotonin and how vital it is for your mood. Serotonin levels in the brain can be assessed using a simple blood test that measures its level within the platelets, which are small particles in the blood. If the level is low, in the clinic we supplement the nutrients that make serotonin. This is the amino acid tryptophan, which then turns into 5-hydroxytryptophan (5-HTP), and then into serotonin. This process requires certain B vitamins, so we usually supplement 5-HTP, tryptophan and the appropriate B vitamins.

How effective is this treatment?

Both tryptophan and 5-HTP have been shown to have an antidepressant effect in clinical trials, although 5-HTP is more effective. There have been 27 studies, involving 990 people to date, most of which proved positive.[33]

So how do they compare with antidepressants? Eleven of the 5-HTP trials were double-blind placebo-controlled, and six of those measured depression using the Ham-D scale. The studies differed in design, so you cannot just add up the scores to get an average, but the improvement rated 13, 30, 34, 39, 40 and 56 per cent. It doesn't take a scientist to realise that these results are a lot better than the average 15 per cent improvement reported for antidepressants.

Are there any adverse effects with 5-HTP?

Some people experience mild gastrointestinal disturbance on 5-HTP, which usually stops within a few days. Because there are serotonin receptors in the gut that don't normally expect to get the real thing so easily, they can overreact if the amount of serotonin is too high, resulting in transient nausea. If this happens, we simply lower the dose. I'll be exploring 5-HTP and other serotonin enhancers in more detail in Chapter 11.

SAMe: your brain's master tuner

There's a process in your brain and body called methylation. There are about a billion methylation reactions every couple of seconds, which help to keep your brain's chemistry in balance. The key nutrient that does all this is called S-adenosyl methionine, or SAMe for short (pronounced 'sammy'). It is a naturally occurring amino acid. You can buy it over the counter in most countries, but not in Europe. It is banned in the EU, not because EU authorities think it doesn't work but because they think it *does* work and have therefore classified it as a medicine. As a medicine it has to have a licence, but since it isn't patentable, no one has a monopoly on it and there's no kind-hearted 'SAMe society' who can raise the kind of money needed to license it. So, in Europe, it's out of the game (see page 122 for more on this 'catch-22' situation). But you can buy it legally over the Internet from abroad. The same fate, by the way, has happened to 5-HTP in Ireland: you can't buy 5-HTP – a naturally occurring nutrient – over the counter because the Irish Medicines Board deems it a 'medicine'. (Ireland is the manufacturing home of a number of large pharmaceutical companies making antidepressant drugs.)

How effective is this treatment?

Over 100 published studies provide well-documented evidence for SAMe's benefit in depression. Many studies show SAMe to be equal or superior to conventional antidepressant drugs. According to one meta-analysis of several of these studies, 92 per cent of patients responded to SAMe, compared to 85 per cent for the tricyclic antidepressants.

Are there any adverse effects with SAMe?

SAMe also has virtually no side effects or withdrawal effects. Occasionally a person experiences mild nausea, much like 5-HTP. For this reason I usually start by giving them 400mg in the morning on an empty stomach, then build it up to a maximum of 1,600mg, but usually 800mg works for most people.

B vitamins balance your brain

The process of methylation, which is needed to make SAMe, also makes other mood-boosting neurotransmitters such as noradrenalin. (If you remember from page 26, the new generation of antidepressants are designed to boost serotonin and noradrenalin levels.) This process depends on a family of 'methylation catalysts'. These include vitamins B_2, B_6, B_{12} and folic acid, as well as another amino acid called TMG. These are often provided together in one supplement designed to support methylation. The measure of methylation, as we'll see in Chapter 13, is your homocysteine level. Homocysteine is a substance in your blood that can predict a person's chances of suffering from a number of illnesses, including depression. A healthy homocysteine level should be below 7. The higher your homocysteine level the more likely you are to feel depressed. This is particularly true for women; for example, a study published in 2003 found that having a level of homocysteine above 15, compared to those with a level below 9, doubles the odds of a woman developing depression.[34]

A high homocysteine level is the best indicator that (a) you are not methylating on all cylinders, so to speak; and (b) you need more of these B vitamins. There are lots of studies showing that giving just one of these B vitamins, such as folic acid, in amounts much higher than the basic RDA (recommended daily allowance) improve your mood. It is sometimes recommended that folic acid be given with antidepressant drugs to enhance their effectiveness. In a study from 2000, comparing the effects of giving an SSRI with either a placebo or with folic acid, 61 per cent of patients improved on the placebo combination but 93 per cent improved with the addition of folic acid.[35]

Folic acid vs antidepressants

How does folic acid, a cheap vitamin with no side effects, compare to antidepressants? Three trials published in 2003 and involving 247 people addressed this question.[36] Two, with 151 participants, assessed the use of folic acid in addition to other treatments, and found that adding folic acid reduced Ham-D scores on average by a further 2.65 points. That's not as good as the results with 5-HTP, but as good, if not better, than antidepressants. These studies also show that more patients treated with folic acid experienced a 50 per cent greater reduction in their Ham-D scores after ten weeks, compared to those on antidepressants.

Fish and the mood-boosting omegas

One of the best single predictors of a country's rate of depression is its fish consumption. In 1998 a survey in the *Lancet* showed that the more fish the population of a country eats, the lower their incidence of depression.[37] Since then many other surveys have found the same thing; for example, among the Greek Islanders, those people eating an extra serving of fish a week almost halved their risk of depression.[38] Even the incidence of homicide [39] and suicide[40] can be predicted from knowing a country's fish consumption. Fish eaters are also less prone to age-related memory loss.

The general assumption is that it's the omega-3 essential fats in fish, specifically carnivorous coldwater fish such as salmon, mackerel and herring, that account for its mood-boosting properties. But fish are also high in other essential nutrients, including vitamin D and phospholipids. One of the main phospholipids, phosphatidyl choline, is also a methyl nutrient, helping those vital methylation processes that seem so critical for healthy brain function. Eggs, by the way, are another source of both phospholipids and vitamin D.

A variety of health-giving properties

There are three main kinds of omega-3 fat: EPA, DPA and DHA. DHA is more important for building the brain, hence it is vital for the foetus during pregnancy. EPA seems to be the most potent natural antidepressant. It's also a natural anti-inflammatory, reducing inflammation within the arteries and the joints, and hence it is good for people with heart disease as well as arthritis. There's also lots of evidence that EPA also reduces aggression[41] and can calm down the mind, so it helps with inflammation of the mind as well as the body.

How effective is this treatment?

To date there have been about 20 trials testing the mood-boosting effects of omega-3 fats. A meta-analysis of 13 of the best-designed trials finds a clear mood-boosting effect of an average of 46 per cent reduction in the depression rating.[42] That's a lot more than you'd expect on an antidepressant drug, and it's without side effects – except for healthier arteries and joints, and smoother skin.

We'll be going into detail on some of these studies to tease out what works best, and for whom. But there's no doubt that taking something like 1,000mg of EPA a day is a good mood booster. Unless you are eating oily fish almost every day, you are unlikely to achieve this kind of level.

In our 100% Health Survey there was little difference in the mood rating between those who had none and those who had one serving of oily fish a week. But those who had two were clearly better off, and those who had three or more even more so. I hedge my bets and eat oily fish at least three times a week as well as supplementing extra omega-3 fish oil every day, and eating a ground seed mix containing both flax, chia and pumpkin seeds, which are rich in the vegetarian form of omega-3, called alpha linolenic acid. Although this type of omega-3 fat isn't nearly as potent as the fish oils, the brain can convert some of it into EPA.

Vitamin D, the sunshine vitamin

Just about everyone feels better when the sun shines. This shouldn't be so surprising since we are, in effect, solar powered, relying on plants to store the sun's energy in carbohydrate, the body's primary fuel. The sun's energy is also stored as vitamin D and essential fats, both found richly in coldwater oily fish. Effectively, sunlight stored in plankton is passed up the food chain, through little fish into carnivorous oily fish.

The Inuit survived, and stayed healthy, due to their diet of seal meat with its high intake of nutrients: seals eat oily fish, and the oils are then stored in their fat and used as an energy source during the winter months (this is essential because they live in the darker regions of the world, which are devoid of sunlight for months on end).

For most of us today, the decline in oily fish consumption, which is largely due to fat phobia created by the popularity of low-fat diets, has fuelled an epidemic of both omega-3 and vitamin D deficiency. This is doubly bad if you live far away from the equator, for example in Britain, where you have little strong sunlight (and with little desire to expose your skin to the sun), for months on end in the winter.

More and more evidence is linking vitamin D deficiency to worsening mood and memory. Although in its early days in terms of research, a few research groups have given vitamin D supplements to those suffering from depression and reported excellent results. I'll be looking at these studies in Chapter 14 so that you can see for yourself the benefits vitamin D supplementation can deliver.

Mood-boosting minerals

Three essential minerals – zinc, magnesium and chromium – which are all deficient in a typical Western diet, are linked to worsening mood.

Rich sources of both zinc and magnesium are found in seeds, nuts and beans. Green leafy vegetables are also an excellent source of magnesium. The decline in consumption of these foods in a typical Western diet may explain the widespread deficiency in those minerals. Chronic stress, a hallmark of 21st-century living, also further depletes these minerals.[43] Few people achieve even the basic RDA levels for these minerals and we frequently find deficiencies when we test patients at the Brain Bio Centre.

Both zinc and magnesium are vital for hundreds of enzyme reactions in the brain and body; for example, they are required for proper methylation, and for making neurotransmitters such as serotonin and noradrenalin. They are also needed to turn essential fats in foods, such as seeds and fish, into prostaglandins, which are thought to be the form in which essential fats do their good.

Magnesium and zinc

The role of magnesium in depression was first discovered in 1921 by P. G. Weston, who used it to help 50 of his patients to relax and sleep.[44] Since then there have been many other studies demonstrating the important role played by magnesium in brain biochemistry and how it benefits mental health.

A study by George and Karen Eby in the US of patients with major depression found that they recovered rapidly, in less than a week, by taking 125–300mg of magnesium with each meal and at bedtime.[45] People who are depressed tend to have lower magnesium levels and there's some evidence that antidepressants help to raise magnesium levels within cells.[46]

Animal studies have shown that animals perk up when given extra magnesium and zinc[47] and that zinc appears to give serotonin levels a boost,[48] which may be how it improves mood. In one study, adding a supplement of 25mg of zinc improved recovery in people with depression who didn't respond to antidepressants.[49]

One of the simple tests we use at the Brain Bio Centre is measuring something called HPL in urine, and it is a good indicator of whether you need more of these minerals.[50] Nutritional therapists often use the urine test to find out if you need more zinc. The RDA of zinc is

10mg, but we find this isn't enough if you tend to feel low. Most people, anyway, are getting less than this from their diet. Supplementing 20mg of zinc, plus 300mg of magnesium a day can make all the difference.

The chromium connection with depression

The essential mineral chromium, despite being known about for 40 years, still doesn't even have an RDA. This means that this vital mineral is often sidelined. But recent studies show some rather remarkable and rapid effects when giving chromium supplements to people diagnosed with 'atypical depression' (more on this in Chapter 7). Chromium is essential for insulin to work properly, but may also affect serotonin in the brain.

In the past, most people who were diagnosed with depression were older, female and skinny, who were not sleeping well, and who had a poor appetite and a consistently flat mood. Nowadays, however, more and more people who are prone to low moods are almost the opposite: overweight, tired all the time, craving carbohydrates and sugar, prone to mood dips and often very emotionally sensitive. These attributes describe 'atypical' depression, even though at least a third, if not half, of people diagnosed with depression fit this bill. These people respond particularly well to chromium, and often lose weight and have reduced sugar cravings as a side effect.

The amount of chromium you need to get this kind of boost is up to 600mcg, which is about ten times more than you are likely to get from food. Chromium is found in whole foods, and refined out of the white stuff; for example, refining sugar removes 98 per cent of the chromium. So stay away from white bread, white pasta, rice and all sugars (because even raw sugar affects your blood sugar level, as I explain in Chapter 7).

A FAST-ACTING IMMEDIATE BOOST

The good thing about chromium, which comes in 200mcg supplements, is that if it is going to work it will do so within days, giving you an immediate boost in mood and a decrease

CONTINUED...

in cravings. The easiest way to find out is just to take two 200mcg tablets with breakfast and one with lunch. If you feel better within three days, keep going. You can always try, after a week, taking two and then one to find the lowest dose that makes a difference. If you don't start feeling perkier within a week, it's unlikely to help you.

How effective is this treatment?

John Docherty, professor of psychiatry at Weill Medical College of Cornell University in upstate New York gave 113 patients with atypical depression either 600mcg of chromium or a placebo for eight weeks and measured them on the Ham-D scale. At the end of the eight weeks, 65 per cent of those taking chromium saw a major improvement in their depression, compared to only 33 per cent on the placebo.[51] In another study, carried out by researchers at Duke University Medical Center, in North Carolina, 70 per cent of those taking chromium improved, with a greater than 66.6 per cent drop in the Ham-D scale compared to none on placebo.[52] This kind of improvement is far greater than antidepressant drugs, again without side effects.

The herb St John's wort

Probably the best-known 'alternative' treatment for mood problems is St John's wort (*Hypericum*). It's not quite in the same category of the nutrients we've been talking about, which so many of us are unwittingly deficient in. You can't really be deficient in St John's wort (or Prozac for that matter), but it appears that St John's wort has many of the benefits of antidepressants, without the long list of frequently reported side effects.

Dr Hyla Cass is one psychiatrist, formerly associate professor at UCLA Medical School in California, who prefers to use St John's wort to antidepressants. She says:

As a psychiatrist, I have prescribed St John's wort for many years, and have found it to be at least as effective as medications, if not more so, and without their debilitating side effects. Rather than simply treating symptoms, St John's wort works with the body's chemistry to treat the underlying imbalance.[53]

How effective is this treatment?

Dr Cass's experiences are borne out by a large body of research over more than 30 years. The results of all this research were published in 2009 involving a total of 29 trials (5,489 patients) including 18 that compared St John's wort with placebos and 17 that compared it with standard antidepressants.[54] In the words of the researchers: 'The available evidence suggests that the hypericum extracts tested in the included trials a) are superior to placebo in patients with major depression; b) are similarly effective as standard antidepressants; c) and have fewer side effects than standard antidepressants.' So, why aren't doctors recommending it? It's more to do with politics and money, than science. We'll be looking more closely at the evidence for St John's wort, and when and how to use it for best effect, in Chapter 15.

In this chapter I've introduced you to some of the most effective natural mood boosters: amino acids, such as 5-HTP and SAMe, B vitamins, omega-3 fats, minerals and St John's wort. In Part 2 you'll discover which of these are most likely to give you a lift, and exactly what to eat and supplement to give you a boost.

Chapter 6

QUICK WINS TO LIFT YOUR MOOD

I hope by now you realise that there is lots that you can do to help boost your mood, enthusiasm and drive – by making changes to your diet, attitude and lifestyle, and by taking supplements. In Part 2, I'll be looking closely at the ten most potent, and proven, ways to improve your mood, and you'll be able to work out which ones are likely to help you the most. Remember, each one of us is different and there is usually more than one factor that is responsible for dampening your enthusiasm.

One of the biggest problems when you are feeling tired and down is that this is also the hardest time to get enough drive and motivation to make the key changes that are going to improve things. Also, when you're feeling down you are more likely to be cynical and sceptical about anything anyone suggests, including me. The good news is that these nutritional changes don't depend on you having a positive attitude about making them. They just require you to make the changes. As you've seen, they work better than placebos and better than conventional drugs. There's also no real concern about side effects. So the only two issues are: (1) making the decision to implement them, and (2) the costs involved.

Working out the costs

Most healthy food is no more expensive than unhealthy food. Yes, fish is more expensive and you might have to add a little extra to your weekly shopping bill to eat oily fish three times a week. Supplements also cost. Once again, fish oils and 5-HTP, my favourite amino acid, are more expensive than basic B or C vitamins. The cost of a decent daily supplement programme is equivalent to the cost of smoking five cigarettes a day plus drinking one glass of wine at home, or less than the cost of a speciality coffee at Starbucks.

There's a basic rule about supplements: the worse your health the more you need, and the better your health the less you need. If your system is significantly depleted you need more to kick-start your brain and body's biology back into balance, and then you need less to maintain it. Most people end up on a maintenance supplement programme after six months. I'll explain how this works and when to cut down in Part 3.

Getting started

For now, just stay focused on the first month, or even the first week, starting today. Most people begin to feel better within a week. So, what can you do right now, starting today? Here are my ten favourite easy options to help you on the road to feeling good:

1 Take a supplement of high-potency EPA (omega-3 fish oil) and supplement twice a day, with food.

2 Take a supplement of 5-HTP 100mg, or St John's wort 300mg, and supplement twice a day, away from food.*

3 Take one 400mg SAMe each morning, then double to two after three days.

4 Try 200mcg chromium, two in the morning and one at lunchtime. This is especially helpful if you crave carbohydrates, or are overweight and tired a lot of the time. If it's going to work you'll feel it within a week.

5 Eat oily fish (salmon, mackerel, herring, kippers, sardines) three times a week.

6 Exercise every day for 15–30 minutes (it's even better if you exercise outside). This could mean a brisk walk every day or joining a yoga class and doing a lengthy session twice a week.

7 Get started on my mood-boosting low-GL diet (see Chapter 17).

8 Find a counsellor or psychotherapist and commit to seeing them once a week.

9 Make an appointment at the Brain Bio Centre, especially if you are having major problems or are on medication (see Resources).

10 Whatever supplements you try, always take a high-potency multivitamin that provides at least 15mcg of vitamin D, 10mg of zinc, 200mg of magnesium, plus 20mg of B_6, 200mcg of folic acid and 10mcg of B_{12}.

***Note** Don't take either 5-HTP or St John's wort if you are currently taking an antidepressant. Read Chapters 11 and 15 for more information on this.

Pick any three of the above ten options and put them into action right now. You can find supplements that combine 5-HTP, chromium, B vitamins and vitamin D – killing a few birds with one stone. This will probably mean a trip to your nearest health-food store or visiting one of the websites listed in Resources.

Also, make a commitment to reading Part 2 of this book over the next week, filling in the questionnaires in each chapter. They are provided to help you find your most effective, personalised Feel Good Factor programme.

Part Two

MY TOP TEN MOOD-BOOSTING SECRETS

In this part I introduce you to my top ten mood-boosting secrets. Each one explains a different factor that can contribute towards low mood and depression, whether caused by imbalances in blood sugar levels, hormones or nutrients, or having insufficient sleep and exercise. I also explain how the mind can become caught up in a repeating pattern of unhappiness. There is much research that has shown how you can correct imbalances through nutrition and a healthy lifestyle, and I also describe ways you can actively help yourself to find, and keep, that Feel Good Factor.

Chapter 7

BANISH THE SUGAR BLUES

If you feel tired a lot of the time and have gained weight, especially around your middle, and if you crave carbohydrates or sweet foods and have lost that Feel Good Factor, there's a good chance that you are losing the ability to keep your blood sugar level even. Learning how to become the master of your blood sugar balance is the secret to having more energy, a better mood and controlling your weight – and losing it if you need to.

Losing blood sugar balance is one of the most common health issues of 21st-century living and eating, and it lies behind the steady increase in obesity, diabetes, heart disease and hormone-related cancers such as breast and prostate cancer. But it's also strongly linked to worsening mood and memory. Loss of blood sugar control, technically called disglycaemia, is one of the signs of a shift in your internal biology, called 'metabolic syndrome'. As well as high blood sugar levels, signs of metabolic syndrome include high cholesterol and insulin resistance, where the body no longer responds properly to insulin, the main hormone that keeps your blood sugar level in check.

The vast majority of people in countries eating a Western diet have degrees of metabolic syndrome without even knowing it; for example, the majority of people who are overweight have insulin resistance, but so do about one in four people who are not overweight and who have apparently normal blood sugar.[55] Have a look at the blood sugar check overleaf. If you score high, the chances are you have insulin resistance too. This is a road you don't want to be on because, ultimately, it leads to metabolic syndrome, weight gain, diabetes and heart disease. I'm going to show you how to switch tracks and, in the process, improve your mood.

Questionnaire: check your blood sugar

		Yes	No
1	Are you rarely wide awake within 15 minutes of rising?	☐	☐
2	Do you need tea, coffee, a cigarette or something sweet to get you going in the morning?	☐	☐
3	Do you crave chocolate, sweet foods, bread, cereal or pasta?	☐	☐
4	Do you often have energy slumps during the day or after meals?	☐	☐
5	Do you crave something sweet or a stimulant after meals?	☐	☐
6	Do you often have mood swings or difficulty concentrating?	☐	☐
7	Do you get dizzy or irritable if you go six hours without food?	☐	☐
8	Do you find you over-react to stress?	☐	☐
9	Is your energy now less than it used to be?	☐	☐
10	Do you feel too tired to exercise?	☐	☐
11	Are you gaining weight, and finding it hard to lose, even though you're not noticeably eating more or exercising less?	☐	☐

Score 1 for each 'yes' answer

Total score: ☐

Score

0–2

Well done! Your blood sugar balance is likely to be good. If you have a couple of 'yes' answers you probably need only to fine-tune your existing diet and lifestyle, rather than making radical changes, to achieve a health benefit. So read this chapter and act on those recommendations that you are not already following.

3–4

You are starting to show signs of poor blood sugar balance and are no doubt suffering as a result. If you don't address the underlying causes now, you will continue to struggle with maintaining stable energy levels and will probably, if you're not already, start to gain weight. Concentrate on cleaning up your diet and follow the supplement advice in Part 3.

5–7

You are almost certainly struggling with poor blood sugar balance, food cravings, fluctuating energy levels and maintaining your weight, as well as worsening mood and memory. If you follow the advice in this chapter, together with the dietary and supplement programme in Part 3, you should soon start to see an improvement in your symptoms.

8 or more

Your blood sugar balance is out of control – but you can reverse the symptoms you are experiencing by following the advice in this chapter and in Part 3. The key challenge for you will be quitting sugary foods and stimulants. As you cut these out of your diet, you will be rewarded with better mood, better energy levels and more stable weight.

Understanding blood sugar

Here's a quick lesson in how your body turns the food you eat into either energy or fat. All carbohydrate foods (bread, cereal, rice, pasta, fruit, sweets, sugar) are digested down into glucose, which then enters the bloodstream. When your blood sugar level goes up, the body squirts insulin (a hormone) into the bloodstream, which takes the glucose out of the blood as quickly as possible, because too much glucose is dangerous. When you have more glucose than you need in the blood, the excess is taken to the liver and rapidly converted into fat, which is then dumped into storage, firstly around your middle.

Every time your blood sugar level goes too high, the glucose damages your blood cells and arteries by sticking to them. This is called glycosylation. Also, if your body continues to make more insulin to lower the sugar highs, over time it becomes more and more insensitive to insulin. The result is that now you have to make even more to get the same effect. The best measure of how often your blood sugar level is peaking is something called 'glycosylated haemoglobin' (or HbA1c), which literally means 'sugar-coated red blood cells'.

The effects of blood sugar that's out of balance

As you lose blood sugar control, you get sugar highs and sugar lows. When your blood sugar is low, you feel tired, irritable, moody and hungry, craving sugar, carbohydrates and stimulants such as caffeine or nicotine. You also make adrenal hormones, called glucocorticoids (or cortisol), which then turn you into a hunter ... for sugar. From an evolutionary point of view, this is what would have motivated our ancestors to go hunting. These adrenal hormones make you more aggressive, impatient, pessimistic and on edge – all good qualities if you are hunting. They also play a major role in controlling your mood.[56]

So, by now you have too many sugar highs indicated by raised glycosylated haemoglobin, insulin resistance and too many glucocorticoids floating around, turning you into a sugar, carb and stimulant junkie (more on the stimulants and caffeine later on). These are the classic hallmarks of metabolic syndrome.

Metabolic syndrome and mood

What's all this got to do with your mood? There is now overwhelming evidence that metabolic syndrome and depression go hand in hand, so much so that a recent review of the evidence in a leading psychiatry journal is headed 'Should depressive syndromes be reclassified as "Metabolic Syndrome Type II"?'[57] If you are not depressed, but have metabolic syndrome, you are twice as likely to have depressive symptoms within seven years, says one study by Finnish researcher Dr H. Koponen.[58] Other studies also show relevant findings: children with metabolic syndrome are more likely to become adults with depression;[59] a study of older Australian men found that those with metabolic syndrome are 137 per cent more likely to be depressed;[60] and a study of Japanese working men found that those with metabolic syndrome more than doubled their chances of experiencing depression – the greater the waist circumference, the greater were the odds of the person being depressed.[61]

Of course, you could argue that being overweight is, itself, depressing, but the association goes both ways. If you are depressed, even if you are not overweight, you also have a much greater risk of developing metabolic syndrome. If you are depressed but don't have metabolic syndrome yet, you are likely to develop it soon.[62] Furthermore, people who are depressed have two-and-a-half times the risk of developing metabolic syndrome within seven years.[63]

Low mood and insulin resistance

If you look at the individual components of metabolic syndrome, you can see the same link with low mood. In a study of Chinese people, aged between 50 and 70, depressive symptoms and insulin resistance went hand in hand.[64] The more depressed you are the higher your glycosylated haemoglobin is likely to be, and vice versa.[65] In fact, the link between depression and blood sugar has been around for a long time. Sir Thomas Willis, the 17th-century medical pioneer who conclusively established the diagnosis of diabetes, noted that 'sadness and long sorrow often precedes this disease'. Two epidemiologists at the Johns Hopkins School of Medicine found that the incidence of diabetes in depressed people is 2.5 times that of the general population. Depression often precedes diabetes by two to three decades. Of course, you could also say that having diabetes is depressing, but people with undiagnosed diabetes double their odds of depression, whereas those actually diagnosed triple their odds.[66]

Whether you are young or old, male or female, Chinese or American, if your blood sugar is out of whack, you are going to be prone to low moods and low energy, with ever-increasing weight, especially around your middle. So, what's the way out? Before I explain this, there's one more thing you need to know and that is why feeling blue often leads to sugar cravings.

Why low mood leads to sugar cravings

I've already spoken about the important amino acid tryptophan – a constituent of protein – and how it's the raw material the body needs every single hour to make serotonin. Low serotonin, as we know, is associated with low mood.

So, when starting off the day, which kind of breakfast would be most likely to increase your brain's serotonin levels and improve your mood? A high-protein breakfast or a high-carbohydrate breakfast?

Logically, one might think that high protein means more amino acids, and more amino acids, such as tryptophan, would mean more serotonin. But the reverse is true. Brain levels of serotonin, and mood, go up after eating *carbohydrate* not protein, even when there's no tryptophan in the food.[67] Although this seems counter-intuitive, there's a simple reason for it.

Tryptophan, the protein constituent from which we make mood-boosting serotonin, is carried from the blood into the brain by insulin, and insulin is *only* released if you eat carbohydrate.

If you crave something sweet when you feel down, and it makes you feel better, the chances are you've unconsciously learned that you need insulin to raise serotonin.

Why low-carb, high-protein diets aren't good for mood

If you are overweight, you may have heard about low-GL diets, which are the state-of-the-art way to lose weight. GL stands for glycemic load and it is a precise measure of what a meal will do to your blood sugar. The basic dynamic is simple: if you can keep your blood sugar level even, you'll have more energy, crave fewer carbohydrates, feel less hungry and lose weight. This approach to weight loss, which is the basis for my book, *The Low-GL Diet Bible*, works much better than conventional low-fat, low-calorie diets[68] because these kinds of diets tend to substitute carbohydrates for fats, so that you will have sufficient to eat.

But there are two ways to achieve a low-GL diet. One is to avoid carbohydrates as much as you can. This we call a high-protein, low-carb diet, typified by the original Atkins Diet. The other way is to eat a bit less carbohydrate and a bit more protein, but to be very choosy about the kind of carbohydrates you eat, choosing the low-GL varieties. This would mean, for example, choosing oats instead of rice- or corn-based cereal, brown rice instead of white rice, berries instead of bananas. This is my kind of low-GL diet: slightly higher in carbs, but choosing those that slowly release their sugar content to avoid big sugar peaks in the bloodstream. But which diet is better for your mood?

Many trials in which people lose weight report improvements in mood. If you look better you'll probably feel better about yourself. But, in a trial comparing the mood-boosting effects of a high-protein, low-carb diet compared to a conventional low-calorie, high-carb diet, the positive benefit of losing weight didn't produce the same long-term improvement in mood for those eating the low-carb diet compared to those on the low-fat, high-carb diet.[69] This, of course, is consistent with the finding that we need some carbohydrate, and some insulin release, to improve mood-boosting serotonin activity in the brain.

Slow-releasing carbohydrate works differently

Would a low-GL diet that gives you slow-release carbs, more akin to the principles of my Holford Low-GL Diet, give better results? An American study put overweight people on a calorie-reduced diet, either with low-GL or high-GL carbs. Both groups lost weight, but those in the low-GL group had much better mood ratings than those in the high-GL group, whose depression rating got significantly worse over time.[70]

We have found the same thing in a small study of 16 people following my low-GL diet over 12 weeks. As well as losing weight and having more energy, half reported fewer symptoms of depression and more stable moods. This is also consistent with the results in our 100% Health Survey of 55,570 people. Sugar-based foods were the biggest predictor of poor mood. A person having three or more servings of sugar-based snacks a day increased their risk of being depressed by over two-thirds.[71]

That's one of the reasons why I advocate a low-GL diet that includes carbohydrate in each meal, albeit slow-releasing carbohydrate. That way you get the weight loss, plus the mood boost, without the high blood sugar levels found in traditional low-fat, low-calorie diets. In Part 3, as part of your mood-boosting action plan, I will show you how to eat a low-GL diet based on three simple rules that are easy to follow whether you are eating at home or out. Beforehand, there's one more piece of the blood sugar balancing equation that's vital for you to know to get an immediate mood boost.

Chromium and 'atypical' depression

It has long been known that supplementing the mineral chromium, usually provided in a 200mcg tablet, helps to stabilise blood sugar. This is because without chromium, insulin (the hormone that carries excess glucose out of the blood into the body and brain) can't work. But thanks to research by Professor Malcolm McLeod from the University of North Carolina, chromium has proved to be not just a vital nutrient for blood sugar stability but also a highly effective antidepressant for those with 'atypical' depression – that is, depressed people who are gaining weight, who feel tired all the time, crave carbohydrates and could sleep forever, unlike the classic 'depressive' type who suffers from a loss of appetite, weight loss and insomnia.[72] In fact, animal studies clearly show that chromium is mood boosting, improving serotonin reception in the brain.[73]

Questionnaire: do you have atypical depression?

		Yes	No
1	Do you crave sweets or other carbohydrates, or tend to gain weight?	☐	☐
2	Are you tired for no obvious reason, or do your arms and legs feel heavy?	☐	☐
3	Do you tend to feel sleepy or groggy much of the time?	☐	☐
4	Are your feelings easily hurt by rejection from others?	☐	☐
5	Did your depression begin before the age of 30?	☐	☐

Score

If you answer 'yes' to even one of these questions and you often feel low, the chances are chromium will help you.

McLeod's discovery happened by chance when one of his patients, George, who had been severely depressed for several years, suddenly recovered completely after taking a nutritional supplement. McLeod thought it was a placebo effect and, since the supplement contained ephedra, a potentially dangerous herb, he asked George to stop taking it. What happened in the following week amazed McLeod. 'It was unbelievable. I didn't believe it at first, but without the supplement his depression returned.' McLeod couldn't ignore the rapid change and concluded that it might be to do with one of six ingredients in the supplement. He then gave George an unidentified envelope containing only one ingredient to take for the next week. Six weeks later, having ruled out ephedra, guarana (which made the depression worse), kava and two other substances, McLeod found that it was the chromium in the supplement that actually worked.[74]

Atypical depression is on the increase

These days, at the Brain Bio Centre, we see as many patients with the symptoms of 'atypical' depression as 'typical' depression. According to McLeod, between a quarter and a half of people diagnosed with depression fit the atypical description. This is confirmed by a survey of several hundred depressed patients, which found that atypical depression affects between 25 and 42 per cent of people with depression, and an even higher percentage of depressed women.[75] So, given the number of people whose tendency to depression falls into this category, 'atypical' is a bit of a misnomer.

McLeod went on to test his theory by running a double-blind study of 15 patients with atypical depression. Five were given a placebo and ten were given 600mcg of chromium picolinate, which is much better absorbed than cheaper forms of inorganic chromium, such as chromium chloride. At the end of eight weeks, seven out of the ten participants taking chromium experienced a major improvement in their depression, compared to none on the placebo.[76]

A larger trial confirms McLeod's finding. One hundred and thirteen patients with atypical depression were given either 600mcg of chromium or a placebo for eight weeks and measured on the Ham-D scale. Sixty-five per cent of those taking chromium saw a major improvement in their depression, compared to 33 per cent on the placebo.[77]

Are high doses of chromium safe to take?

Chromium is a remarkably safe mineral even at levels 100 times higher than above. McLeod gave 3–5mcg per 450g (1lb) of body weight, and sometimes more for people with diabetes. Some people need this amount to stay free from depression. George, McLeod's original patient, has been taking chromium for a decade and it has positively transformed his life. McLeod recommends taking it twice a day, although you should take it in the morning (at breakfast and lunch), as it can occasionally cause insomnia and vivid dreaming.

Because chromium levels decline with age, the older you are the more you need. Our diets are generally very deficient in this mineral anyway, but the more fast-releasing carbohydrates you eat, the more chromium you will lose. Stress also depletes chromium.

How does it compare with antidepressants?

According to McLeod, chromium is far superior to SSRIs because it has no side effects. Even if its ability to relieve symptoms of depression is only half as powerful as an SSRI, chromium is better for this reason. It is also much faster acting than SSRIs, usually working in just two to three days, whereas SSRIs can take several weeks to produce relief. Furthermore, chromium often reduces symptoms much more effectively than SSRIs. McLeod has found that many of his patients had complete relief in a matter of weeks just by taking it. The Ham-D scores of several patients dropped below 5 within two weeks, which means they were no longer depressed. You don't see this on SSRIs.

Chromium and other nutritional treatments

These results with chromium fit in well with other promising frontiers in the nutritional treatment of depression. The amino acid 5-HTP, which is the precursor of serotonin, needs insulin to get from the blood into the brain. So chromium, which is essential for insulin to work, might be playing a leading role in this process (see Chapter 11). Omega-3s also improve serotonin reception (see Chapter 10). Given the role that stress, caffeine and highly refined and high-sugar diets have on blood sugar, and the lack of chromium and omega-3s in most people's diets, it isn't perhaps so difficult to comprehend why the incidence of depression is on the increase in the 21st century.

In Part 3 I will explain exactly how to put into action what I have discussed in this chapter, specifically all about my mood-boosting low-GL diet, and when and how to supplement chromium.

SUMMARY

- Eat protein with carbohydrate.
- Choose low-GL foods.
- Have three low-GL meals and two snacks a day.
- Stay away from very sweet and sugary foods.
- Supplement chromium – at least 200mcg a day, up to 600mcg if you fit the description of atypical depression.
- See Part 3 for your complete Mood-boosting Action Plan.

Chapter 8

BALANCE YOUR HORMONES

An extremely common cause of feeling low in mood, motivation and energy is an underactive thyroid. Now, this may or may not apply to you, but it is certainly worth checking out. In the US, thyroid medication is the fourth most commonly prescribed drug. Ten times more women are affected than men and, in the UK, an estimated one million women are affected, making it more common than diabetes.

The thyroid gland is situated in the base of the throat, just below the Adam's apple. It makes the hormone thyroxine, which tells all the brain and body cells to keep active. Too much and everything goes too fast: you lose weight, you can't sleep and your heart races. Too little and your system slows down: fatigue, dry skin and constipation are the classic symptoms. Often, as a long-term consequence of stress and sub-optimum nutrition, the thyroid gland can start to underproduce thyroxine. This is a classic cause of depression and lethargy, although symptoms of irritability, anxiety and panic attacks have also been reported in those with low thyroxine levels. Other telltale signs of an underactive thyroid are poor memory or concentration, indigestion or constipation, haemorrhoids, skin problems, feeling cold and not tolerating heat well, fluid retention and weight gain.

Do you have an underactive thyroid?

Some thyroid experts think that symptoms are as important as tests for an underactive thyroid, but ideally you want both. Complete the thyroid check below. If you do have a lot of these symptoms it is well worth getting your thyroid tested.

Questionnaire: check your thyroid

	Yes	No
1 Do you feel the cold and go around turning up the heat, to the annoyance of others around you?	☐	☐
2 Are you troubled by excess heat as well as cold, but you don't sweat much?	☐	☐
3 Do you find it hard to get up in the morning, and do you drag yourself around for an hour or so before getting going?	☐	☐
4 Do you have noticeably less drive and vigour than you used to?	☐	☐
5 Do you have difficulty losing weight?	☐	☐
6 Do you have unexplained fluid retention that makes you look puffy?	☐	☐
7 Do you suffer from constipation?	☐	☐
8 Do you suffer from excessive flatulence?	☐	☐
9 Do you suffer from depression and/or have you been diagnosed with depression?	☐	☐
10 Are you always forgetting appointments and names or things you have planned to do?	☐	☐
11 Has your hair become fine and wispy, and is it thinning and falling out constantly?	☐	☐
12 Have you lost the outer third of your eyebrows, and are your eyelashes disappearing?	☐	☐
13 Do you suffer from repeated cystitis or kidney infections?	☐	☐
14 Do you suffer from repeated upper respiratory tract infections?	☐	☐
15 Have you have lost your libido?	☐	☐
16 Do you have a family history of hypothyroidism?	☐	☐

Score 1 for each 'yes' answer

Total score: ☐

Score

Less than 5
It is unlikely you have a thyroid problem.

5–10
Do the thermometer test below. If this is positive, get your thyroid function checked.

11 or more
There's a good chance that you do have an underactive thyroid. Do the thermometer test below. If this is positive, have your thyroid function checked and see a nutritional therapist. Remember, symptoms are as important as a thyroid test. If you have symptoms but your thyroxine result is low–normal, you may still have a problem.

THERMOMETER TEST

Because thyroxine speeds up your metabolism, which produces heat, the definitive symptom is a drop in body temperature. This is something you can check yourself by taking your temperature with a thermometer. (**Note**: women should do this test on day two or three of their period, as body temperature fluctuates during the menstrual cycle.) Here's how you do it:

1 Before you go to bed, shake out a thermometer and keep it by your bed.

2 When you wake in the morning, and before getting up, put the thermometer under your arm and lie there for 10 minutes. Your basal temperature should be 36.5–36.7°C (97.7–98.1°F).

3 Do this for at least two days.

4 If either of your temperature readings are below 36.5°C (97.7°F), take it again over a longer period, say a week, to see if it is low on a fairly regular basis. If it's lower than 36.5°C (97.7°F), you probably have an underactive thyroid.

If you suspect you have a thyroid problem, your doctor can run a blood test to investigate this possibility further.

What happens when the thyroid is underactive?

When the body is making too little thyroxine it triggers a hormone produced in the brain, called thyroid-stimulating hormone (TSH). A high level of TSH is the most common basis for diagnosis, but different countries and experts use different cut-off points. The 'official' line in the UK is that the normal TSH level is between 0.5 and 5, even though some experts don't treat unless the TSH level is over 10. The American Association of Clinical Endocrinologists recommended that 'doctors consider treatment for patients who test outside a TSH range of 0.3 to 3'. Thyroid expert Dr Leonard Wartofsky from Washington Hospital Center in the US thinks an upper level of 3 may even be too high. 'According to the latest thinking, the upper level should be about 2.5,' he says. 'My UK colleagues say there's no evidence that treating below 10 is beneficial but I'd say it was mixed; studies showing benefit are coming in. We certainly see dramatic improvements in patients treated within reference levels.'

So, if you do get your thyroid tested, make sure you get a copy of the actual results. As well as measuring TSH you'll get a measure of two kinds of thyroxine called T4 and T3. T4 is converted into T3, which is the active hormone, so if you have a normal level of T4 but a low level of T3, you may not be converting the thyroxine your body makes into the active T3. If this is the case, follow my nutritional guidelines below; however, an apparently normal thyroxine level, if at the low end of normal, backed up by lowered temperature and symptoms, may still be worth treating.

The causes of an underactive thyroid

A quite common cause of an underactive thyroid is that your body is producing what are called anti-thyroid antibodies. Some research groups find that more than half of those with underactive thyroids have anti-thyroid antibodies[78] so this really is something that should be tested. This can also be tested as part of a thorough thyroid test (see Resources for good private laboratories used by nutritional therapists). If you test positive, it means that you have an autoimmune disease where your body is mistakenly attacking cells that produce thyroxine. A common cause of this is an unidentified food allergy, which I'll be discussing in the next chapter. Many people, for example, who are unknowingly allergic to wheat gluten (called coeliac disease), produce anti-thyroid antibodies. Once the offending food allergen is identified and avoided the thyroid can return to normal function. This is thought to happen because the body's immune system cross-reacts, attacking both the offending food protein and the thyroid gland.

If your TSH is high but your thyroxine levels (T4 and T3) are normal, one possibility is that you have too much oestrogen, which competes with thyroxine at hormone receptor sites. In other words, your body is able to make thyroxine, but the message isn't getting through. (I discuss this further later in the chapter.)

Treating an underactive thyroid

Although the medical approach is to give you thyroxine, which I'll discuss shortly, this hormone is made from the amino acid tyrosine. Tyrosine is converted into thyroxine and then into T3 by enzymes that depend on zinc, selenium and iodine. B vitamins are also important for a process called 'methylation' (see Chapter 13) required for the production of thyroxine. So, I suggest you start by taking a high-strength multivitamin that contains iodine, zinc (at least 10mg) and selenium. You could also try adding extra zinc (up to 20mg a day in total) or extra selenium (up to a maximum of 200mcg in total). Kelp is a good source of iodine, as is seafood.

Swollen thyroid, or goitre

If you have an underactive thyroid gland and it is swollen, causing a goitre, this can be a sign of iodine deficiency. You need about 1,000mg of tyrosine (some people need twice this), taken on an empty stomach. Tyrosine is, itself, a mood booster for some people (see page 116 in Chapter 11).

Help from a healthy diet

Most of all, put yourself on a strict low-GL diet, as explained in Part 3, eating lots of fresh fruit, vegetables and whole-foods, and minimise stress and stimulants (such as caffeine and nicotine). You may also want to supplement 200mcg of chromium, as this often helps to lift low energy and a low mood. This total strategy sometimes even reverses borderline low thyroid function.

Act on allergies

If you have discovered that you have an allergy (explained fully in Chapter 9), you will need to avoid that food for at least three months. Once the offending food allergen is identified and avoided the thyroid can return to normal function. It is believed that the body's immune system cross-reacts, attacking both the offending food protein and the thyroid gland.

CASE STUDY: JENNIFER

Jennifer had suffered with depression on and off since she was 16. She was diagnosed as having severe depression and was given various antidepressants, all of which aggravated her symptoms. By the time she came to the Brain Bio Centre she was finding it very hard to cope with everyday life and was experiencing suicidal thoughts, anxiety and extreme lethargy, both mentally and physically. She had put on 19kg (3st/42lb) in weight due to cravings and binge eating. Her tests revealed that she had very high levels of anti-thyroid antibodies, as well as several food intolerances, and low levels of B vitamins and essential fats.

Three months after starting her allergen-free diet and taking supplements, Jennifer said she was 'thrilled' at how well she was doing. Her mood had lifted considerably and she had lost 7.7kg (17lb). A few months later she went back to work full-time, something she had feared would never happen.

CASE STUDY: FELICITY

Felicity was diagnosed with clinical depression in 2006. Given the choice between hospitalisation and medication, she began taking antidepressants, which caused awful side effects. When she came to the Brain Bio Centre in 2008 she complained of physical and mental lethargy, mood swings, nervousness, suicidal thoughts and insomnia, and was overweight. Tests revealed she was deficient in omega-3, had low noradrenalin levels and vitamin D (more on this later) and that her thyroid function was sub-optimal.

Felicity started on a supplement regime that supported her thyroid, addressed her deficiencies of omega-3 fats and vitamin D and corrected the imbalances in neurotransmitters, while also supporting her general health. She also switched from snacking on refined-sugar foods to low-GL snacks of fruit with nuts or seeds.

Cut back on dairy foods

As explained at the beginning of the chapter, if your TSH is high, but your thyroxine levels (T4 and T3) are normal, one possibility is that you have too much oestrogen. Because eating a lot of dairy products can promote excess oestrogen, reduce or exclude dairy from your diet, but do increase nuts or seeds to make sure you get enough calcium.

The homocysteine link

It is also worth checking out your homocysteine level with a simple pinprick home test kit, if your doctor won't do it for you (I explain all about homocysteine in Chapter 13). This is because there is a direct link between low thyroid hormone and high homocysteine. Homocysteine itself indicates how efficient your body is at a process called methylation, which depends on B vitamins and helps to make hormones. If your homocysteine level is high, it means you need more B vitamins.

Research from all over the world – from the US and UK to the Czech Republic, Denmark and France – has reported the link between homocysteine and thyroid problems. Danish scientists have found that the higher your homocysteine level, the lower your thyroxine level is likely to be, and the greater the likelihood that you will experience symptoms and signs of an underactive thyroid. So they now recommend that anyone with a high homocysteine score be routinely checked for thyroid problems.[79]

Endocrinologists at the Cleveland Clinic Foundation and the University of California, Davis, have also found that hypothyroidism is often associated with high homocysteine levels. Following drug treatment to normalise the thyroid, homocysteine levels also returned to normal.[80]

I'll be talking much more about high homocysteine in Chapter 13, because this alone is a common reason for feeling low. Giving extra B vitamins often returns homocysteine, thyroxine and TSH levels to normal. Two of the vitamins required for normal methylation and a normal homocysteine level are the B vitamins folic acid and vitamin B_{12}. These are often found to be low in those people who have an underactive thyroid. According to one research group 40 per cent of people with underactive thyroids are B_{12} deficient, if tested, and feel much better once given extra B_{12}.[81]

All the above steps can help to correct fundamental deficiencies and reverse endocrine burnout, which is perhaps the most common cause of an underactive thyroid. But if none of this works, I'd recommend exploring the possibility that you may benefit from a low dose of thyroxine. With the right nutritional support, the chances are you won't need very much to feel a lot better.

Synthetic thyroxine or armour thyroid?

If your doctor is prepared to treat you, you will almost certainly be offered eltroxine, a synthetic version of T4, which the body then turns into the useable form T3. (That's why a test for just T4 can be misleading, because if your problem is that T4 is not being properly converted into T3, it won't be spotted – you will have plenty of T4 and may still feel terrible.)

Some people don't respond well to doses of T4, so a few doctors are prepared to offer an older form of treatment known as armour thyroid. This is a dried extract of pig thyroid, which was used regularly on the NHS back in the 1960s. Mainstream doctors will say that T4 is more consistent in quality and lacks the risks associated with treating with animal extract, but its supporters claim that, chemically, armour thyroid is more like the human hormone and that some patients do very well on it. It is no longer licensed in the UK but can be obtained from the US, and doctors can issue a private prescription for it. Some nutritional therapists also use glandular extracts. In any case you are going to have to seek the advice of a professional to obtain any thyroid extracts.

If you'd like some help interpreting your test results or getting your nutritional programme right, I recommend you see one of my nutritional therapists (see Resources). The best place to find a list of sympathetic doctors is through one of these two patient support groups: Thyroid Patient Advocacy-UK and Thyroid UK (see Resources).

Oestrogen and progesterone deficiency and menopausal mood swings

Low moods are particularly common during the menopausal phase. Many women experience depression, anxiety, insomnia and worsening memory. In one survey, 45 per cent of women experienced minor depressive symptoms during the menopause, whereas 27 per cent complained of nervousness or irritability.

Vitamin B_6, zinc, magnesium and essential fats all greatly help to reduce menopausal symptoms and allow the body to better adapt to changing hormonal levels. Serotonin deficiency is also very common in menopausal women, who often benefit greatly from additional tryptophan or 5-HTP (see Chapter 11).

Menopausal depression is often the result of oestrogen and progesterone deficiency. According to John Lee, a doctor from California who pioneered research using 'natural' progesterone, mood, mental clarity and concentration frequently improve with the use of transdermal progesterone skin creams. Most conventional HRT includes synthetic progestins, sometimes called progestogens. These do not work so well and they've also been linked to an increased risk of breast cancer.[82]

The good thing about natural progesterone is that the body can also make oestrogen from it; however, that being said, some women find greater relief with both oestrogen and natural progesterone therapy. The combination of the two prevents the cancer risks associated with unopposed oestrogen.

The andropause and depression in men

The effects of testosterone deficiency are not unlike the effects of oestrogen and progesterone deficiency. Around a third of men in the

40–69 age group complain of a range of symptoms that commonly include, in order of importance, loss of libido, erectile dysfunction (inability to get or maintain an erection), depression and worsening memory and concentration. These are the classic symptoms of the andropause or male menopause.

Despite years of research, pioneered in Britain by Dr Malcolm Carruthers, who wrote *The Testosterone Revolution*, many doctors still deny the existence of the male menopause; however, these symptoms, especially depression, should be taken seriously. Depression in men is harder to diagnose, since men tend to get angry rather than sad. Supplementing the hormone testosterone can help the symptoms of andropause.

If the symptoms sound like the ones you have, it is well worth having your testosterone levels measured. If low, meaning below 12 nmol/l, then you may benefit from testosterone replacement therapy; however, symptoms are as important, if not more so, than testosterone levels in the blood. This is because most testosterone in the blood is not 'free', but bound and unavailable. The free testosterone is much harder to measure. Salivary testosterone levels may be a better indicator, backed up by symptoms. You can test your symptoms and have a salivary testosterone test (see Resources). The salivary test also measures your DHEA levels (see below). These tests are also available through nutritional therapists.

Supplementation for low testosterone

If you have low testosterone, supplementing extra can really help. Dr Elizabeth Barrett-Connor studied 680 men aged between 50 and 89 and found a direct relationship between testosterone levels and mood.[83] In the UK, Dr Carruthers has treated 1,500 men and found a consistent elevation in mood once testosterone levels become normal.

From a nutritional point of view, make sure you are eating adequate protein and a low-GL diet. Essential fats are required for healthy sperm and prostate function, antioxidant nutrients protect testosterone from being destroyed, and zinc helps everything to do with male sexual health and hormonal balance, so make sure you are getting enough of all these nutrients. If you follow the Feel Good Factor regime in Part 3 you will have all the nourishment you need.

DHEA deficiency and adrenal exhaustion

Sometimes mood swings and depression can be a result of too much stress and adrenal exhaustion. The adrenal glands, which are on top of the kidneys, produce a number of hormones: cortisol, adrenalin, noradrenalin and DHEA. Prolonged stress can result in an inability to produce sufficient amounts of these motivating molecules. DHEA levels are frequently found to be low in anxious and depressed people, and have been associated with aggressive and cynical attitudes and the loss of enjoyment of life. Without sufficient adrenal hormones, especially DHEA, you lose your 'get up and go' and your ability to cope with the normal stresses of life, becoming more anxious, on edge and depressed. Of course, the answer is to decrease your stress levels, but how do you get your adrenal function up to scratch?

The answer can be to supplement DHEA. A study in 1997 gave depressed, middle-aged and elderly people 30–90mg of DHEA and found a clear improvement in their mood.[84]

I never recommend DHEA, from which the body can make other adrenal hormones, without first running a saliva test to determine whether someone has low levels of this hormone. If they are low, I recommend 25mg a day for women and 50mg a day for men until these levels are normalised. DHEA isn't available over the counter in Britain but it is in the US. You can buy it by mail order for your own use. A nutritional therapist can determine your DHEA levels.

Testing for hormonal imbalances

If you suffer from mood swings and depression, but if basic changes to your diet, including taking supplements, hasn't helped, you can check for hormonal imbalances quite simply. A saliva test can measure your oestrogen, progesterone, testosterone and DHEA levels. These tests are available through nutritional therapists who will then advise you about how to bring your hormones back into balance.

SUMMARY

- If you have the symptoms associated with an underactive thyroid, test your body temperature.
- If it is low, get your thyroid tested. You can also test other hormone imbalances with a hormone saliva test.
- If your results indicate low or borderline levels, go on a strict low-GL diet and supplement 500mg or 1,000mg of tyrosine on an empty stomach or with a carbohydrate snack twice a day. Start off with the lower dose. Also, take a high-strength multivitamin containing at least 200mcg of folic acid, 10mcg of B_{12}, plus iodine, zinc and selenium. You can also try kelp tablets for a month, which are a good source of iodine.
- Make sure your daily supplement programme provides at least 20mg of vitamin B_6, 10mg of zinc and 200mg of magnesium.
- Test your homocysteine and, if high, follow the guidelines in Chapter 13 to lower it.
- Discuss with your doctor or health professional using thyroid glandular extracts rather than synthetic thyroxine, if this doesn't make you feel much better. If your oestrogen, progesterone or testosterone levels are low, consider supplementing natural, or 'bio-identical', hormones.
- See Part 3 for your complete Mood-boosting Action Plan.

Chapter 9

HAVING THE GUTS TO BE HAPPY

When you feel tired, depressed, stressed or anxious, the chances are you wouldn't consider that your digestive system, or a food you've eaten, could have anything to do with it. But the gut and our emotions are linked. In the same way that nervousness can upset the tummy, so foods that don't 'agree with us' can upset our mind. Most strong emotional feelings are felt physically somewhere along the digestive tract. We feel them in our gut and often experience them affecting our appetite and our ability to digest properly.

Your second brain

Science is discovering that the digestive system acts like a 'second brain' producing neurotransmitters, such as serotonin, hormones and immune-transmitters, called cytokines, that literally cross-talk with the brain. These cytokines have receptors on the immune cells and the brain cells. We now know that every emotion you experience has a direct biological effect, affecting your nervous, digestive, endocrine and immune systems.

Your 'second brain' also reacts every time you eat a piece of food. The gut lining, which makes up a surface area about the size of a tennis court and the thickness of half a sheet of paper, is the interface between you and your food, and it is programmed to react against anything eaten just in case it is a foe. Ninety-nine per cent of the time, the job of a healthy immune system – which is more active in the gut than anywhere else – is to switch off that reaction so you can enjoy the food you're eating without your body fighting it. That switching-off mechanism can be assisted by increasing your intake of omega-3 fats, found in fish and seeds, such as flax and pumpkin seeds.[85] These essential fats not only stop the gut becoming inflamed but they also stop psychological inflammation – in other words, the feelings of aggression, irritability and depression, the latter of which is sometimes anger turned inwards. I'll be explaining about this role of essential, or 'happy', fats in detail in the next chapter.

Weight and stress increase food reactions

If you are overweight, diabetic or insulin resistant, or if you have some level of stress, you are more likely to react against the food you eat, inhibiting its proper digestion and absorption. Likewise, if your gut has suffered a degree of damage – perhaps through the regular use of alcohol or painkillers, or through bloating, gut infection or antibiotics – you are also more likely to react against the food you eat. The average person in Britain takes over 300 painkillers a year and the common ones, such as aspirin and ibuprofen, are the gut's worst enemies, because they damage it, making you more prone to allergy.

The simple amino acid, glutamine, which feeds the gut mucosa, helps to heal a damaged gut. So, if you think your gut is in need of repair, try taking a heaped teaspoonful of glutamine powder in water before bed each evening for one week, or look out for a combination formula that contains nutrients to aid gut healing (see the supplement section in Resources). Eating a digestion-friendly diet that minimises potentially allergenic foods can also help (I explain further about allergies later in this chapter).

Communicating with the outside world

Because of the gut's connection with the brain, any gut-related problem has a direct effect on the brain. The gut is the interface between the exterior world and your body, and our experience of life is the interaction between the exterior world, which is perceived through our senses, and how we interpret them. It makes sense, therefore, that your gut and your brain would be talking to each other.

There is a nerve that connects the brain and gut directly, called the vagus nerve, but other systems in the gut also communicate. When you have inflammation – either in the gut or elsewhere – such as an aching joint or IBS, cytokines tell your brain to put you into 'retreat' mode and to take time out. It's all part of a normal evolutionary reaction. When you're sick, injured, stressed or down, you want to effectively retreat into your 'cave' to recover your strength so that you can face the world. Allowing your gut to recover is an important part of keeping it healthy and promoting good digestive and mental health, as I will explain. Likewise, if you are feeling stressed, your gut is directly affected, making your digestive system less tolerant to those foods that you may be mildly intolerant to.

Cytokines, activated by gut reactions, can make you feel depressed and have direct effects on the mood-boosting neurotransmitter serotonin (see Chapter 11 for more on this). In fact, a healthy gut is essential for producing the vast majority of serotonin made in the body.

The role of gut bacteria

Our gut bacteria also affect our mood. We have more bacteria in the gut than cells in our entire body, and they are absolutely vital for proper immunity. Probiotics (which are supplements of good bacteria) help to promote and 'train up' cytokines to do their job properly. In so doing they not only calm down inflammation in the gut but they also help signal to the brain to calm down, reducing stress reactions. Probiotics also boost something called 'brain-derived neurotrophic factor', which makes the brain's receptors more responsive to neurotransmitters. Research has found that supplementing probiotics has been shown to improve mood in those who are prone to depression.[86] (I'll be talking about the brain's feel-good neurotransmitters in the chapters that follow.)

When you go into a state of stress, hormones communicate this to the gut, which then shuts down the digestion and promotes inflammation, which could manifest as anything from a headache to an aching joint or gut ache. This has been studied, for example, when baby rats were separated from their mother.[87] However, research has found that giving probiotics reduces this stress response and helps to reset the system out of stress.[88]

Taking probiotics helps to reduce levels of adrenal hormones and, by reducing inflammation, switches your body away from a reactive state. Digestive enzymes also help to do this.

Finding the right probiotics

When taking probiotics, it's very important to have the correct 'human strains', which are identical to the strains that naturally reside inside us. The two essential probiotic families are called *Lactobacillus acidophilus* and bifidobacteria. The most effective way to restore a healthy balance of gut bacteria is to take supplements that contain millions of bacteria rather than probiotic drinks, which are usually loaded with sugar.

Why wheat might be a problem

Certain foods are particularly bad news for the gut. One of these is wheat. It contains a protein called gluten, which is largely composed of a substance called gliadin. This substance irritates the gut and often causes an allergic reaction. Once you are allergic to wheat your immune system produces antibodies, and these attack wheat proteins every time you eat them. Even though wheat has become a staple food in our modern diet, it is actually a very new food to the diet of humans. Our ancestors, when they first started cultivating grains a few thousand years ago, ate very little wheat compared to today. (The same is true for dairy products, which are the most common allergy-provoking food.)

Coeliac disease is often undiagnosed

The most severe form of wheat allergy is called coeliac disease, where the wheat protein wears away the gut lining, thereby affecting the body's ability to absorb nutrients. Coeliac disease is vastly under-diagnosed and a common cause of depression. There is a strong genetic aspect to this condition. If you have a mother, father, brother or sister with coeliac disease, you have a one in ten chance of having it too, which means you have a 30 times higher risk than the average person.

Medical textbooks still wrongly say that coeliac disease occurs in only one in 5,000 or so people. Owing to remarkable advancements in laboratory screening, however, we have learned that it occurs more frequently than ever imagined. More recent studies appearing in the *Lancet* medical journal have reported a prevalence of 1 in 122 of the Irish, 1 in 85 of the Finnish and 1 in 70 of the Italians in northern Sardinia.[89]

Coeliac disease is thought to be such a health threat in Italy that the government has considered mandating that all children, regardless of whether they are sick or not, must be tested for gliadin sensitivity and coeliac disease by six years of age. In Britain we are still in the Dark Ages in terms of recognising the widespread prevalence of the disease.

The other medical myth about coeliac disease is that a doctor should be able to diagnose it easily from symptoms, even though the condition is rarely seen. Doctors are told that the signs and symptoms, mostly emanating from the abdomen, are unmistakable: chronic diarrhoea/episodic diarrhoea with malnutrition, abdominal cramping, abdominal distention or bloating, weight loss, and so on. Doctors are told to expect to hear complaints of weakness, fatigue and loss of appetite; however, an exceedingly common symptom of coeliac disease is depression, but this is not on the list of recognised symptoms.[90]

However, you don't have to have coeliac disease or gut damage to react to wheat gluten. It can simply cause neurological problems such as depression, headache or migraine.[91] This is another example of the gut–brain link.

How allergies can affect the brain

Most people don't think of food allergies as a potential cause of tiredness, low mood, poor concentration, anxiety or even more severe conditions such as schizophrenia. Yet it has been known for a very long time that allergies to foods and chemicals can adversely affect mood and behaviour in susceptible individuals. Food allergies have been proven to cause a diverse range of symptoms, including: chronic fatigue, slowed thought processes, lack of motivation, irritability, agitation, aggressive behaviour, nervousness, anxiety, depression, alcoholism and substance abuse, schizophrenia, hyperactivity (ADHD), panic attacks, autism and varied learning disabilities.[92]

Early studies into allergy and mental health

A doctor from Munich, Joseph Egger, was one of the first pioneers studying the link between allergy and mental health. He decided to test 30 patients for allergy, who were suffering from anxiety, depression, confusion or difficulty in concentrating. The study used a double-blind placebo-controlled trial, by giving the patients either dummy foods, or their allergenic foods, in small quantities, disguised so that they didn't know what they were eating. The results showed that the food allergens alone were able to produce severe depression, nervousness, feelings of anger without a particular object, loss of motivation and severe mental blankness. The foods that produced the most severe mental reactions were wheat, milk, cane sugar and eggs.[93]

Another pioneer of food and chemical sensitivity was Dr Benjamin Feingold, whose Feingold Diet became famous in the 1970s. He investigated the possibility of food allergies and sensitivity to salicylates (found in aspirin) in 96 patients diagnosed as suffering from alcohol dependence, major depressive disorders and schizophrenia, compared to 62 control subjects selected from adult hospital staff members. The results showed that the group of patients diagnosed as depressives had the highest number of allergies: 80 per cent were allergic to grains, and all were allergic to egg white. Only 9 per cent of the control group were found to suffer from any allergies.[94]

These studies are prime examples of how problems created by allergies can often produce a multitude of mental as well as physical symptoms, because they affect the central nervous system, and even the whole body. The state of inflammation potentially induced by an allergic reaction is found in many mental-health conditions including depression[95] and is probably one of the main mechanisms by which a food allergy affects the brain. What's more, allergies are very specific to the individual, as are the symptoms they create, so any diagnosis can only be made individually by proper food allergy testing.

Testing for allergies

At the Brain Bio Centre we routinely test individuals with low mood or motivation for allergies. It is not at all uncommon for us to find that putting a person on the allergy-free diet they need relieves symptoms of depression, insomnia or anxiety. So, if you suffer from poor concentration, insomnia, anxiety or other symptoms of depleted mental health, it's well worth investigating whether food allergies are playing a part.

If your score is high on the following questionnaire there's a good chance you have food allergies.

Questionnaire: check your food sensitivity

	Yes	No
1 Do you suffer from allergies?	☐	☐
2 Do you suffer from IBS?	☐	☐
3 Can you gain weight in hours?	☐	☐
4 Do you get stomach pains or bloating sometimes after food?	☐	☐
5 Do you sometimes get really sleepy and tired after eating?	☐	☐
6 Do you suffer from hay fever?	☐	☐
7 Do you suffer from excessive mucus, a stuffy nose or sinus problems?	☐	☐
8 Do you suffer from rashes, itches, eczema or dermatitis?	☐	☐
9 Do you suffer from asthma or shortness of breath?	☐	☐
10 Do you suffer from headaches or migraines?	☐	☐
11 Do you sometimes get depressed or have 'brain fog' for no clear reason?	☐	☐
12 Do you suffer from intermittent joint aches or arthritis?	☐	☐
13 Do you suffer from colitis, diverticulitis or Crohn's disease?	☐	☐

	Yes	No
14 Do you suffer from other aches or pains that come and go?	☐	☐
15 Do you get better on holidays abroad, when your diet is completely different?	☐	☐
16 Do you use painkillers most weeks?	☐	☐

Score 1 for each 'yes' answer

Total score: ☐

Score

5 or more

It is well worth exploring the possibility of a food allergy, either by excluding suspect foods for a trial period or having an IgG food intolerance test (see Resources).

It's not all in the mind

Some so-called health experts are sceptical about food intolerances, claiming that they are all in the mind. An example of this is a recent study from the Institute of Medicine at the University of Bergen. They found that, in a group of people self-reporting food hypersensitivity, 89 per cent had irritable bowel syndrome (IBS) and 57 per cent tested positive for a psychological problem – anxiety and depression being the most common.[96] They ran serum tests for a type of antibody called IgE, and also took skin-prick tests and provocation tests, which also involve IgE-based antibody reactions, and found no real correlation. Of course, you can interpret these results in two ways. Either you say that all the people tested are crazy and that IBS is also 'in the mind', or that there's a common underlying cause for both IBS and psychological symptoms.

The convention is that food allergy is caused by the release of IgE antibodies which target the offending food. IgE-based allergies usually produce rapid symptoms and are therefore quite easy to observe by provocation testing: giving a suspected offending food and noticing a reaction in the next hour or so. That's what this study did, and only 8 per cent reacted to one or more foods. You'll probably know if you have an IgE-based food allergy because you normally get quite pronounced symptoms such as asthma, eczema, diarrhoea or vomiting within an hour of eating the food. But there's another kind of antibody called IgG that doesn't always cause immediate reactions and may explain 'hidden' or delayed food allergies. In the case of IBS, there is no difference between the number of IgE antibodies in those with IBS versus those without, but there is a big difference in IgG antibody levels.[97] IBS sufferers were much more likely to have high IgG levels to wheat than to other foods.

To test further whether these IgG-based food sensitivities were an actual cause of IBS, researchers at the University Hospital of South Manchester devised an ingenious study. They tested 150 IBS patients using YorkTest's IgG-based food allergy test. The patients' doctors were then given real or fake allergy test results, without either the patient or their doctor knowing, and the patients then followed what they thought was their allergy-free diet. Only those following their real allergy-free diet significantly improved, and the closer they stuck to the diet the better were the results; however, for those on the sham diets the degree of compliance made no difference. Compared to patients given the commonly prescribed drug Tegaserod, those following the allergy-free diet were seven times more likely to benefit.[98]

Other studies confirm the findings

In one survey of over 5,000 people who had taken an IgG food intolerance test and avoided their suspect foods, more than three out of four reported a noticeable improvement in their condition, with 68 per cent feeling the benefit within three weeks of following the diet. Of those who rigorously followed the diet, 76 per cent showed a noticeable improvement in their chronic symptoms. For those with psychological symptoms, the response rate was 81 per cent, and for those with gastrointestinal complaints, such as IBS, the response rate was 80 per cent. However, for those with depression, 92 per cent responded to the allergy-free diet and for those with panic attacks (15 people) all benefited. On reintroduction of the offending foods, 92.3 per cent felt a return of symptoms.[99] So, the chances of it working for you if you have these kinds of symptoms are very good indeed. (If you'd like to know more about the scientific evidence for food allergies and intolerances see www.patrickholford.com/foodallergyevidence.) See Resources to find out how to get yourself tested.

CASE STUDY: PETER

> When Peter came to the Brain Bio Centre he had a long history of mental-health problems, which left him unable to work, and over the years he'd tried various antidepressants. He had suffered with periods of severe depression and sometimes experienced suicidal thoughts, along with many unpleasant side effects from the medication. He felt he wanted to be able to 'enjoy life to the full' but wasn't able to.
>
> When we tested him for IgG-based food intolerances he reacted to many foods, including gluten, egg white, corn and barley. After removing these foods from his diet, and following a supplement programme to support his general health, he began to experience fewer spells of feeling down and noticed what he described as a 'huge improvement' in his general well-being and mood.
>
> Peter did experience a bad patch while he was on holiday, when his symptoms started to return. He had strayed from his usually healthy diet and was eating a lot of the foods he was intolerant to, but as soon as he got his diet back on track he almost immediately began to feel better again. He has now started working and feels that he has accomplished his goal of enjoying life.

Most food allergies aren't for life

The more severe and immediate IgE allergies last for life, but these are less common than the IgG intolerances. In the latter case, if you remove the offending item strictly for four months, and then heal the gut with a combination of glutamine, digestive enzymes and probiotics, you can lose your sensitivity to that food.

Once you've found out what you are allergic to, and avoided it strictly for four months, you can reintroduce these foods, one at a time, waiting for 48 hours to see if you have a return of any of your symptoms. If you do not, then reintroduce the next food. You can also reduce your likelihood of developing an allergy by 'rotating' foods – which means eating them no more frequently than every four days. This is a good idea if you have a history of reacting to a certain food such as wheat or milk. If you do react, assume that you are still allergic to the food. But, before then, it's best to 'heal' the gut as previously explained.

SUMMARY

Next time you're feeling stressed or low, think about your digestive system:

- Have you been eating allergy-promoting foods? It might be worth getting yourself tested.
- Are you lacking in omega-3 essential fats from oily fish, flax and pumpkin seeds? (There's more on this in the next chapter.)
- Have you been drinking alcohol or taking painkillers, or have you taken a course of antibiotics?
- Might you benefit from taking some probiotics, glutamine and digestive enzymes? These are available in combination in some supplements and are worth taking for a month to help restore gut health (see the supplement section in Resources).
- See Part 3 for your complete Mood-boosting Action Plan.

If you want to know more about allergies, read *Hidden Food Allergies* by Patrick Holford and Dr James Braly (Piatkus).

Chapter 10

WHY OMEGA-3 FATS ARE ESSENTIAL

There's a lot that can be learned from the past. One example is the discovery that there is a difference between the earliest human skulls found in Africa along the coast, compared to those found inland. The ones inland had more dents in them: the meat-eating inlanders, it appeared, hit each other on the head more that the fish-eating coastal dwellers. The same principle appears true today. Extraordinary as it may sound, you can actually predict a country's murder rate[100] as well as its depression[101] and suicide rate[102] simply by knowing its seafood intake. That's what Commander Joe Hibbeln, chief psychiatrist for the US navy, discovered when he pooled the data from numerous countries.

In Britain, as the intake of omega-3 has declined, and omega-6 from margarine and processed foods has increased, so too has the murder rate.[103] This data is rather 'hard' in the sense that different people have different ideas about what defines a diagnosis of depression or aggression, but murder and suicide are rather indisputable. In the graph overleaf you'll see that Bulgaria is not a great place to live in this regard, while Norway, Japan and Hong Kong are much better choices.

Wonderful seafood

So, what is it about seafood that boosts your mood? Seafood is the best source of essential fats, which are found in incredibly high concentrations in the brain. These fats are also one of the most potent mood-boosting 'drugs' when supplemented in concentrated capsules. The dry weight of your brain is 60 per cent fat, so perhaps it shouldn't be

Fish consumption and incidence of homicide

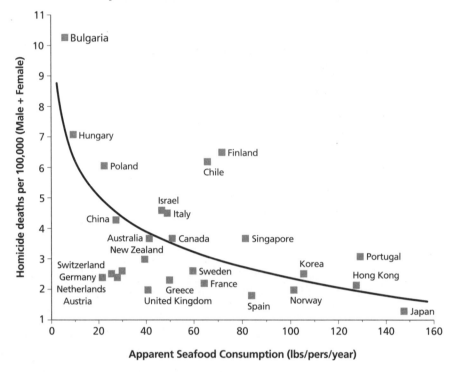

J.R. Hibbeln, *World Review of Nutrition and Dietetics*, 2001;88:41–46
(used with the kind permission of the author)

such a surprise to find that we all depend on a daily intake of essential fats.

So essential are these fats that if a pregnant woman is deficient in them, her growing baby will rob her brain so that it can grow its own – it's a case of 'Mummy, I shrank your brain', and one of the reasons why many pregnant women feel forgetful and prone to depression. Among pregnant women, the lower the intake of omega-3s the higher their chances of becoming depressed.[104]

A lack of fish or fish oil is also linked to increasing hostility and aggression.[105]

The truth is that most people don't get enough essential fats. But before we get into the nuts and bolts of what they do, where you get them from and which ones to use for a mood boost, let's take a look at your signs and symptoms with the essential fat check below.

Questionnaire: check your essential fats

		Yes	No
1	Have you ever suffered from skin rashes, eczema or dermatitis?	☐	☐
2	Do you suffer from dry or rough skin?	☐	☐
3	Do you have dry hair or dandruff?	☐	☐
4	Do you experience joint stiffness?	☐	☐
5	Would you describe yourself as generally anxious or hyperactive?	☐	☐
6	Do you suffer from depression?	☐	☐
7	Do you get irritable or angry easily?	☐	☐
8	Do you generally feel apathetic and unmotivated?	☐	☐
9	Do you have difficulty concentrating or easily become confused or distracted?	☐	☐
10	Do you have a poor memory or difficulty learning?	☐	☐
11	Do you have cardiovascular disease?	☐	☐
12	Do you have high blood lipids (cholesterol or triglycerides)?	☐	☐
13	Do you have an inflammatory disease such as eczema, asthma or arthritis?	☐	☐
14	Do you take painkillers most weeks?	☐	☐
15	Do you rarely eat oily fish (mackerel, salmon, sardines, fresh tuna); for example, once or less a week?	☐	☐
16	Do you rarely eat raw nuts and seeds; that is, less than every other day?	☐	☐
17	Do you eat fewer than four eggs a week?	☐	☐
18	Do you have two or more alcoholic drinks most days?	☐	☐
19	Do you eat fried, crispy, burned or browned foods most days?	☐	☐

Score 1 for each 'yes' answer

Total score: ☐

Score

0–2

Congratulations! You don't seem to have any symptoms associated with lack of essential fats (although the ideal score is '0'). However, you could still benefit from reading this chapter and introducing the recommendations that you are not currently already following, to safeguard yourself in the future.

3–4

There is room for improvement and you are likely to benefit from a little extra help in this area. Follow the recommendations in this chapter and Part 3.

5–7

You are likely to be lacking essential fats and suffering as a consequence. Follow the advice in this chapter, making sure that your diet is the best that it can be, and follow the supplement programme in Part 3.

7 or more

It is extremely unlikely that your current diet is providing enough essential fats to meet your needs for optimal health. Follow the advice in this chapter and in Part 3, which includes increasing your intake of essential fats both from food and from supplements.

Getting to know your omegas

As you can see from the illustration opposite, there are two kinds of essential fats: omega-3 and omega-6. Omega-6 fats are prevalent in the oils of seeds of plants that grow in a hot climate. So, sunflower seeds and sesame seeds are full of them. You can think of these oils as storehouses of the sun's enlightening energy.

Omega-3 and -6 fats

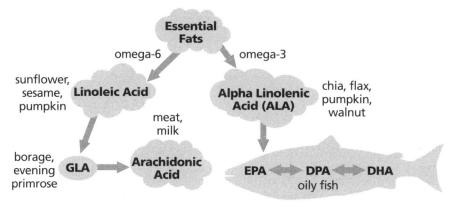

If you live in the northern hemisphere, with not enough light to keep you in bright spirits, nature has invented a rather ingenious way of giving you what you need. In colder water the plankton – made of tiny organisms that absorb and run off the sun's energy – grows in abundance. Little fish live off this. Bigger fish, or rather carnivorous fish with teeth, live off the little fish, and seals live off the carnivorous fish such as mackerel and salmon. As you move up the food chain from krill to seals, the omega-3 fats become concentrated in the flesh. That's why these fish are known as 'oily' fish. And they are literally part of the food chain that brings the sun's enlightening energy up into the northern hemisphere.

Omega-3 fats and the brain connection

Although you can get a type of omega-3 fat called alpha-linolenic acid in vegetation, such as chia, flax and pumpkin seeds, by far the most potent omega-3 fat is EPA, which turns into DPA then DHA. These are the 'Three Musketeers' that not only keep your brain healthy, but also your heart.

These musketeers are not just essential for building and rebuilding your brain but they're also very much part of the equation for happiness. The higher your blood levels of omega-3 fats, the higher your levels of serotonin are likely to be. The reason for this is that omega-3 fats help to build receptor sites as well as improving reception itself. According to Dr Joseph Hibbeln, whom we met earlier, 'It's like building more serotonin factories, instead of just increasing the efficiency of the serotonin you have.'[106] A recent survey in Norway found the same thing. Those who consumed cod liver oil, another rich source of omega-3, had the lowest incidence of depression, and the longer a person had been taking it the less likely they were to be depressed.[107]

Research has confirmed the benefits of fish oils

There have been ten good-quality double-blind controlled trials to date giving fish oils rich in omega-3s to depressed people. In five of them, the findings showed significant improvement, greater than that reported for antidepressant drugs.[108] Most studies on antidepressant drugs report something like a 15 per cent reduction in depression ratings. Three studies on omega-3s reported an average reduction of 50 per cent[109] – and that's without side effects. One of the first placebo-controlled trials, by Dr Andrew Stoll from Harvard Medical School, gave 40 depressed patients either omega-3 supplements or a placebo and found a highly significant improvement in the patients on supplements. In the next study, 20 people suffering from severe depression, who were already taking antidepressants but were still depressed, were given either a highly concentrated form of omega-3 fat – ethyl-EPA – or a placebo. By the third week the depressed patients taking ethyl-EPA were showing major improvement in their mood, whereas those on placebo were not.[110] So you don't have to wait long for a result.

A more recent trial gave a concentrated form of EPA or a placebo to 26 depressed people with bipolar disorder (formerly known as manic depression) and again found a significant improvement in those taking the EPA.[111] Of those studies that used the Ham-D scale, including one recent 'open' trial that did not involve the use of placebos, the average improvement in depression was approximately double that shown by antidepressant drugs, without the side effects. Fish oil supplements have also been shown to help those with depression in pregnancy[112] and those in states of psychological distress[113] but are not always effective in those who experience more 'manic' or anxious states.

Keeping the levels up

So how do the omega-3s do it? It may be because these essential fatty acids help to build your brain's neuronal connections as well as the receptor sites for neurotransmitters. So the more omega-3s in your blood the more serotonin you are likely to make, and the more responsive you will become to its effects, which, as you'll see in the next chapter, is good news. The higher your intake of omega-3s the lower your homocysteine level, an indicator of methylation, is likely to be. The better you are at methylation, a process that depends on B vitamins, the more able you are to make neurotransmitters such as serotonin. In Chapter 13 I'll be explaining why this is good news for your mood.

To achieve a therapeutic amount of EPA of around 1,000mg, you will need to take something like three 1,000mg fish oil capsules a day, ensuring the EPA provided in them adds up to a total of 1,000mg; or take two a day plus three servings of oily fish a week. I always take an essential omega-3 and -6 capsule twice a day and also eat oily fish three times a week. If you do the same, you would only need one extra EPA-rich fish oil capsule, if you feel low, to achieve an average of around 1,000mg of EPA a day.

Cholesterol and your brain

Part of the fat that makes up your brain is, in fact, cholesterol, and that might explain why very low intakes of fat or cholesterol can lead to depression, as seen in a study of 121 healthy young women and anxiety.[114] An eight-year Finnish study of 29,000 men aged 50 to 69 found that those reporting depression had significantly lower average blood cholesterol levels than those who did not, despite a similar diet.[115]

The best dietary way to ensure adequate cholesterol and essential fats is to eat coldwater fish such as herring, fresh tuna (in moderation; see Not All Oily Fish are Equal on page 100), salmon, sardines and mackerel. It remains to be seen whether the current trend of putting millions of people on statin drugs, which are designed to lower cholesterol, will induce a tendency to depression as a side effect. It is not uncommon to be put on these drugs after a heart attack, even if the person's cholesterol level is already low. This might well increase the chances of depression.

Beneficial side effects

Unlike antidepressants, all the side effects of taking in more omega-3 fats are beneficial.

- Oily fish and omega-3 fish oil switch off inflammation caused by eating the wrong foods[116] and fish oil supplements decrease pain and stiffness in arthritis sufferers more effectively than pain-killing drugs.[117]
- Eating oily fish and/or supplementing omega-3-rich fish oil lowers your risk of heart disease[118] and effectively halves the risk of a second heart attack. Doctors in the UK are now recommended to prescribe it to patients after a heart attack.[119]
- Having more omega-3s also gives you flexible, soft and velvety skin; better concentration; reduced addictive cravings, anxiety, aggression and PMS, and less pain.

The Three Musketeers: EPA, DPA and DHA

So far, we've focused on EPA, a specific type of omega-3, largely because most trials have used a concentrated form of this, called ethyl-EPA, which is available on prescription. But in oily fish you'll find three different kinds of omega-3: EPA, DPA and DHA. EPA is more 'functional', meaning that the prostaglandins made from it seem to be the most potent, reducing inflammation or improving mood. On the other hand, DHA is 'structural', meaning that the brain is built from it. The DHA level in a child at birth predicts their speed of thinking at age eight, so DHA is more important in pregnancy and is usually also added to formula milks for babies. But there is a third musketeer, DPA, which few people are aware of, although this may be the most potent omega-3 fat of all.

As you move up the food chain, from plankton to krill (the tiny crustaceans baleen whales feed on), to sardines, salmon, seals and the Inuit, the kind of omega-3 fats change. Algae in the sea that plankton feed off contains only ALA (see illustration on page 95). Sardines contain mainly EPA but, like most fish, are low in DPA. But salmon, mackerel, and especially seals, are exceptionally rich in DPA. So too is breast milk – and the Inuit. Originally, many of the now proven benefits of omega-3 fats were discovered by analysing the diet of the Inuit, which contains a lot of seal and salmon. Despite their very high intake of fat and cholesterol, their risk of cardiovascular disease is minimal. In fact, the higher your level of DPA, the lower your risk of heart disease.[120]

As you can see from the illustration on page 95, ALA (the vegetable source of omega-3) converts into EPA, then EPA into DPA, then DPA into DHA. So DPA sits in the middle of the other two musketeers. It can be converted into either EPA or DHA, so it's highly flexible.

When you eat an oily fish such as salmon, you are getting all three omega-3 fats. Most fish oil capsules provide EPA and DHA but little, if any, DPA. Ideally, you want to supplement all three.

The best fish

There is more to fish than omega-3s. In fact, many surveys show that fish consumption overall, not just oily fish, predicts mood; for example, a survey of older people in Greece found that for every serving of fish a person's chances of having a low mood score halved.[121] Although oily fish are the richest source of omega-3 fats and vitamin D, both of which are associated with a mood boost, all fish provide other nutrients, including B_{12}, a commonly deficient mineral, and phospholipids, which are a major component of the brain. I'll be talking about why these other nutrients are an important part of the Feel Good Factor in later chapters.

In our 100% Health Survey of 55,570 people, the association between improved mood and oily fish consumption only became apparent once a person was eating two or more servings a week. Although it may not be environmentally correct, with declining levels of fish in the sea and an increasing population, the optimal intake of oily/carnivorous fish is probably three to five servings a week. The National Institute for Health and Clinical Excellence (NICE), which advises NHS policy in the UK, recommend all heart attack patients eat two to four portions of oily fish (herring, sardines, mackerel, salmon, tuna and trout) a week. Other surveys have also reported improved mood and less incidence of depression in those eating more oily fish.[122]

Not all oily fish are equal

Have a look at the chart opposite and you will see that the level of omega-3s are a fraction in canned tuna compared to fresh. This is probably because the oil may be squeezed out, and perhaps sold to the supplement industry, leaving a drier meat that is then canned in vegetable oil. In the US you can buy tuna in its own oil. It tastes completely different and much better. So don't rely on canned tuna to provide your omega-3 quota, always try to use fresh fish.

Another problem with oily fish is the potential for mercury contamination, particularly in very large fish such as tuna. This is particularly relevant for pregnant women, since mercury is a neurotoxin and can induce birth defects. I would recommend tuna no more than once a fortnight during pregnancy and a maximum of once a week otherwise. (Yellow-fin tuna has much less mercury than blue-fin tuna.) The same advice applies to marlin or swordfish (though the exact levels are unconfirmed). See the chart below. The best all-rounders are wild salmon, mackerel, sardines, herrings or kippers, which have the highest amount of EPA. The level of omega-3 in farmed salmon will depend upon what they are fed.

A small serving of salmon or mackerel will give you at least 1.5g of omega-3 fats, which is about the bare minimum you need in a week. In pregnancy, women who achieve this have better mood ratings than those who don't.[123]

In terms of EPA, mackerel and salmon are good choices, but the best is herring or kipper, providing almost 1g per serving. The all-time best source of EPA is caviar, providing a staggering 2.7g per 100g, but you'd be pushed to eat, or afford, that much! Any fish roe, and oysters, are also good sources.

Bear in mind that studies in people with diagnosed depression show improvement at intakes of 1g of EPA a day – the amount in a serving of mackerel or salmon. If you eat oily fish three times a week, that leaves four days to supplement, or 4g a week. That's about 600mg a day if you even it out over seven days.

How much omega-3, EPA and mercury is there in oily fish?

Fish Source FSA 2004	Omega-3 g/100g	EPA g/100g	Mercury mg/kg	Omega-3/ mercury ratio
Canned tuna	0.37	0.23	0.19	1.95
Trout	1.15	0.25	0.06	19.17
Herring	1.31	0.90	0.04	32.75
Fresh tuna	1.50	0.09	0.40	3.75
Canned/smoked salmon	1.54	0.47	0.04	38.50
Canned sardines	1.57	0.47	0.04	39.25
Fresh mackerel	1.93	0.65	0.05	38.60
Fresh salmon	2.70	0.69	0.05	54.00
Swordfish	2?	0.13	1.40	1.43?
Marlin	2?		1.10	1.83?

How much to supplement?

I generally recommend, as a basic supplemental level for everyone, about 250mg a day of EPA (or EPA + DPA) or 600mg of total omega-3s (EPA+DPA+DHA). I take a capsule of EPA+DPA+DHA, as well as GLA (omega-6) twice a day, which provides these kinds of levels. If you are feeling low, I recommend topping up with an EPA-rich omega-3 fish oil to achieve the 1g a day. These can provide 300–400mg per 1,000mg capsule. (See Resources for examples.) This will give you about 1,000mg of EPA, including what you achieve from eating fish.

For vegetarians and non-fish eaters

What if you don't like fish or are vegetarian? Non-fish eaters will need to supplement an additional EPA-rich fish oil supplement. Many vegetarians are willing to compromise and take the fish oils. If you are not, and are depressed, there is no vegetarian source of EPA. Instead, you must have two tablespoons of chia or flax seeds a day, or two teaspoons of their oil. Chia is the richest source of ALA. But even this will not give you anything like 1,000mg of EPA, because only about 5 per cent of ALA is converted into EPA. This conversion is dependent on B vitamins and zinc, so supplementing a high-potency multivitamin will definitely help.

SUMMARY

- Eat oily fish three times a week.
- Supplement, twice daily, a capsule of essential omega-3 and -6 oils, providing around 250mg of EPA+DPA.
- Supplement an additional EPA-rich omega-3 fish-oil capsule providing at least 300mg of EPA when you are feeling low.
- See Part 3 for your complete Mood-boosting Action Plan.

Chapter 11

RESTORE YOUR BRAIN'S NATURAL BALANCE WITH AMINO ACIDS

As you may remember from Chapter 4, I explained how SSRI antidepressants give you more of one of the feel-good chemicals in the brain, serotonin, by blocking the brain's ability to break it down, and the same applies to noradrenalin with the use of the newer SNRI drugs. Serotonin is associated with low mood, whereas noradrenalin is associated with a lack of motivation.[124] However, these drugs have an awful record of side effects and not much evidence of benefit, especially for mild depression. Since serotonin and noradrenalin are made from food, specifically amino acids – which are the building blocks of protein – in this chapter I am going to show you how to optimise your ability to make your own neurotransmitters, and restore balance naturally without any side effects. This chapter explores the different ways you can help your body to make enough of its own serotonin and noradrenalin.

The seven main reasons for serotonin deficiency

Women are three times as prone to low moods as men. Many theories as to the reason why have been proposed, some psychological and some social, but the truth is that women and men are biochemically very different. The research of Mirko Diksic and colleagues at McGill University in Montreal demonstrates this. They developed a technique using PET neuro-imaging to measure the rate at which we make serotonin in the brain.[125] What they found was that men's average synthesis rate of serotonin was 52 per cent higher than for women. This, and other research, has clearly shown that women are more prone to low serotonin. In women, low serotonin is associated with depression and anxiety, whereas in men, low serotonin is related to aggression and alcoholism. One possibility is our social conditioning: men 'act out' their moods, whereas women are more conditioned to 'act in' their moods. It's an example of depression being the flipside of anger.

In the last few years we have learned that there are seven main reasons for serotonin deficiency:

1 Not enough oestrogen and/or progesterone (in women); not enough testosterone (in men)
2 Not enough light
3 Not enough exercise
4 Too much stress, especially in women
5 Lack of tryptophan
6 Not enough catalyst vitamins, minerals and essential fats
7 Blood sugar imbalances

Before we go further, complete the serotonin check below to see if you have the kinds of symptoms associated with low levels of serotonin:

Questionnaire: check your serotonin levels

	Yes	No
1 Do you suffer from insomnia?	☐	☐
2 Do you always wake up early in the morning?	☐	☐
3 Do you find it hard to relax?	☐	☐
4 Do you wake up at least two times during the night?	☐	☐
5 Do you find it hard to fall asleep when you've been awakened?	☐	☐
6 Are you often sad or depressed?	☐	☐
7 Do you ever have suicidal thoughts?	☐	☐

	Yes	No
8 Are you often anxious and easily irritated?	☐	☐
9 Have you been under a lot of stress?	☐	☐
10 Have you become less interested in sex?	☐	☐
11 Do you crave carbohydrates when you are low?	☐	☐
12 Do you drink alcohol almost every day?	☐	☐

Score 1 for each 'yes' answer

Total score:

Score

0–2

Well done. You are unlikely to be low in serotonin.

3–4

You have enough symptoms to consider the possibility that you may be low in serotonin. If so, following the supplement advice in this chapter and in Part 3 may help you.

5–7

You have enough symptoms to make it probable that you have low serotonin levels. Follow the advice in this chapter and the supplemental 'extras' in Part 3.

8 or more

You have more than enough symptoms to suggest low serotonin levels. Ideally, get your level checked (see page 113) and follow the advice in this chapter and the supplemental 'extras' in Part 3.

The hormone connection

Hormone imbalance, as we discussed in Chapter 8, is a common contributor to low serotonin; low oestrogen means low serotonin and therefore low moods.[126] This is because oestrogen blocks the breakdown of serotonin. This may largely explain why women are more prone to depression pre-menstrually and during the menopause and thereafter. Low testosterone has a similar effect in men.

Light stimulates oestrogen, but most of us don't get enough of it, as I have already mentioned. (There's more about this in Chapter 14.) There is a massive difference in the light exposure we receive when we are outside compared to indoors, and most of us spend 23 out of 24 hours a day indoors. This exposes us to an average of 100 units (called lux) of light a day, compared to 20,000 lux outside on a sunny day and 7,000 lux on an overcast day. Of course, light deficiency is worse in the winter. Today, more than ever before, many of us rarely expose ourselves to direct sunlight, and certainly not enough to maximise serotonin production.

Stress also rapidly reduces serotonin levels; in contrast, physical exercise improves stress response, and therefore reduces stress-induced depletion of serotonin.

Each of these reasons for serotonin depletion affects women more than men. Men produce serotonin twice as fast as women, allowing them to rebalance it from any of these serotonin depleters, without suffering prolonged blues, provided there's enough tryptophan in their diet. Let's now look more closely at tryptophan, because it's the building block of serotonin.

Essential tryptophan

As you can see in the illustration opposite, serotonin is made from a constituent of protein: the amino acid tryptophan.

Tryptophan is essential for good mood, as researched by Dr Philip Cowen from Oxford University's psychiatry department. He wondered what would happen if you deprived people of tryptophan, and he gave 15 volunteers who had a history of depression, but were currently fine, a nutritionally balanced drink that excluded it. Within seven hours, 10 out of 15 noticed a worsening of their mood and started to show signs of depression. On average they jumped three points on the Ham-D scale.[127]

Tryptophan is the building block for serotonin

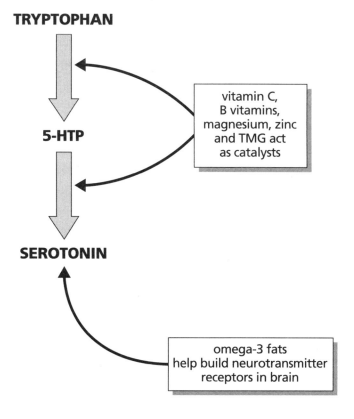

So, does the reverse also apply? If a depressed person takes tryptophan will their mood improve? The answer is yes. Supplementing tryptophan is well proven to improve mood, and it is available on prescription exactly for that purpose. Donald Ecclestone, professor of medicine at Newcastle's Royal Victoria Infirmary in the UK, reviewed the available studies and concluded that supplementing tryptophan leads to an increase in the synthesis of serotonin in the brain, improving mood as effectively as some antidepressant drugs.

How much should you take?

You need about 1g for low mood, and up to 3g a day for actual depression, taken either on an empty stomach or preferably with a carbohydrate food such as fruit, since carbohydrates help its absorption. (Remember that in Chapter 7 we learned that tryptophan needs insulin, from carbohydrate, to be carried into the brain.) Tryptophan also promotes sleep, so it's generally best taken before bed.

Foods rich in tryptophan

Fish, turkey, chicken, cheese, beans, tofu, oats and eggs are particularly rich in tryptophan. As well as supplementing it, it is a good idea to make sure your diet gives you at least 1g a day by eating any two of the following meals, each giving you 500mg of tryptophan.

FIVE WAYS OF EATING 500MG OF TRYPTOPHAN

- Oat porridge made with soya milk, plus two scrambled eggs
- Baked potato with cottage cheese and a tuna salad
- Chicken breast, potatoes au gratin (sprinkled with breadcrumbs and cheese) and green beans
- Whole-wheat spaghetti with a bean, tofu or meat sauce
- Salmon fillet with quinoa and lentil pilaf, and a green salad with yoghurt dressing

---

However, we don't just need tryptophan for making serotonin. It's an essential amino acid for making body proteins such as muscle – and the more muscle mass you have the more able you are to burn fat, helping you to lose excess weight.

Why carbohydrate is important

Eating a meal containing tryptophan doesn't raise brain levels of tryptophan unless you eat it with some carbohydrate. The reason for this anomaly is that tryptophan in the bloodstream competes very badly with all the other amino acids in protein, so little gets across into the brain; however, when you eat a carbohydrate food, such as a potato, this causes insulin to be released into the bloodstream, from which it carries tryptophan into the brain. That's one of the reasons my mood-boosting diet, based on low-GL principles, always combines protein with carbohydrate (as seen in the box opposite).

This may be why depressed people instinctively crave sweet foods to give them a lift. This causes a surge of insulin, which carries tryptophan into the brain, causing serotonin levels to rise. So, if you find sugar gives you a mood lift, you are probably low in serotonin. The trouble is, most carbohydrate snacks are high in refined sugar and fat, and make you fat, which is depressing. The solution is to supplement tryptophan with carbohydrate, and preferably a low-GL carbohydrate. In Chapter 7 you learned that eating protein with low-GL carbohydrate is one of the ways to balance your blood sugar, as well as promoting healthy serotonin levels. This not only improves your mood but it will also reduce your appetite, especially for sugary foods. That's why tryptophan can also help you to lose weight.

The tryptophan controversy

So why don't we generally supplement tryptophan? Thousands of people did, up to 1989, with tremendous results both for depression and for promoting sleep (see Chapter 12). And, in doses of 1,000–3,000mg, it worked.

But in 1989, disaster struck. Hundreds of people taking tryptophan supplements mysteriously developed a condition called eosinophilia-myalgia syndrome (EMS), resulting in 37 deaths. Tryptophan was immediately withdrawn from the market. A long and thorough investigation determined that the culprit was a contaminated or altered tryptophan molecule that contained something called 'peak x'. The contamination occurred when a Japanese company used a new production technology that involved genetically altering a yeast to produce tryptophan. It was one of the first blunders of genetic modification, resulting in unexpected deaths. The mystery was solved.

Despite this finding, however, tryptophan remained banned in the US and many other countries. At ION, we started searching through every reported case of EMS and proved to the British government that they could all be linked to the contaminated batch of tryptophan – thus showing that the pure amino acid tryptophan is not at all toxic. In fact, despite the ban on tryptophan supplements, drug companies in the UK and the US have continued to sell prescription forms of tryptophan and no cases of EMS have been reported.

Thanks to the ION report, the British government rescinded the ban on tryptophan in the UK, quite rightly, on the condition that companies could sell only pure, pharmaceutical-grade tryptophan; however, they also argued that, because the average dose of prescribable tryptophan given by doctors was 2,200mg and since this was clearly 'medicinal' (meaning effective) because it had been prescribed, they would limit the amount in supplements to a tenth of this: 220mg. This limitation was not made on the basis of any safety concerns whatsoever. In fact, 220mg is less than you get in two eggs or a serving of lentils. So, you are going to have to take a lot of tryptophan pills to get up to the effective dose of around 2,000mg. A better solution is to supplement a more effective kind of tryptophan called 5-HTP, as explained below.

5-HTP: the shortcut to serotonin

Although supplementing tryptophan itself has proven an effective blues buster, even more effective is a type of tryptophan that is one step closer to serotonin (see illustration Tryptophan is the Building Block for Serotonin on page 107). This is called 5-hydroxytryptophan, or 5-HTP for short, and it is derived from an African plant called griffonia. The first study proving the mood-boosting power of 5-HTP was carried out in the 1970s in Japan, under the direction of Professor Isamu Sano of the Osaka University Medical School.[128] He gave 107 patients 50–300mg of 5-HTP per day, and within two weeks, more than half experienced improvements in their symptoms. By the end of the four weeks of the study, nearly three-quarters of the patients reported either complete relief or significant improvement, with no side effects. This study was repeated by other researchers who also found that 69 per cent of patients improved their mood.[129]

As already explained on page 43, 27 studies have shown that people who supplemented 5-HTP achieved overall better results in a decrease in depression symptoms compared to those achieved by using antidepressant drugs, with a fraction of the side effects.

In a double-blind trial involving 34 depressed volunteers either the SSRI antidepressant fluvoxamine or 300mg of 5-HTP were given. At the end of the six weeks, both groups of patients experienced a significant improvement in their depression, with those taking 5-HTP having a greater improvement in their depression, anxiety, insomnia and physical symptoms.[130]

Although previous studies had shown 5-HTP to be as effective as the tricyclic antidepressant imipramine,[131] in this study 5-HTP had outperformed an SSRI antidepressant. Given that 5-HTP is less expensive and produces significantly fewer side effects, it is extraordinary that psychiatrists virtually never prescribe it, despite plenty of scientific evidence that it helps to restore normal mood and normal serotonin levels.[132]

How much 5-HTP should you take?

The recommended dosage of this natural supplement, available in any health-food store, is 50–100mg of 5-HTP, twice a day, for depression. In studies, amounts above 300mg a day are not generally more effective.

Unlike tryptophan, it doesn't compete with other amino acids to be absorbed into the bloodstream. In fact, it is very well absorbed, with about 70 per cent of what you eat being absorbed into the bloodstream and much of that crossing into the brain.[133] Unlike tryptophan, 5-HTP is not so essential to take with a carbohydrate snack, although there is some evidence that this might help a little. If you are serotonin deficient, the brain is perfectly able to synthesise more from 5-HTP.

Vitamins that boost 5-HTP

Look again at the illustration, Tryptophan is the Building Block for Serotonin, on page 107, and you'll see that the conversion of tryptophan into 5-HTP, and then into serotonin, requires a whole lot of catalyst nutrients. An enzyme called hydroxylase (not shown on the illustration) converts tryptophan into 5-hydroxytryptophan. This enzyme also needs vitamin C to work properly, so making sure you get enough from both diet and supplements helps to optimise your serotonin levels.

Vitamin B_6 is a vital part of the chemical process that converts 5-HTP into serotonin, so you need to take about 20mg of B_6 for every 100mg of 5-HTP.

You'll also see that tryptophan can be used by the body to make vitamin B_3 (niacin). By supplementing a little extra vitamin B_3, more tryptophan becomes available to make serotonin effectively because you've already made sure you have enough B_3. Niacinamide, in this respect, is the best form of B_3 to take. Later on, when we look at the importance of sleep, we'll be talking about how your brain makes melatonin from serotonin and therefore from tryptophan or 5-HTP. This conversion requires the B vitamins B_6, B_{12} and folic acid, as well as zinc and magnesium. You can think of all these B vitamins as oiling the wheels of the processes that turn the food you eat into mood-boosting neurotransmitters.

Are there any side effects with 5-HTP?

Supplementing 5-HTP has been shown to be effective in treating a wide variety of conditions, including fibromyalgia, binge eating associated with obesity, reduced sugar craving, weight gain, chronic headaches and insomnia, as well as depression. That's the up side.

What about potential downsides? In some sensitive people, antidepressant drugs can induce an overload of serotonin called 'serotonin syndrome', characterised by feeling overheated, with high blood pressure, twitching, cramping, dizziness and disorientation. Some concern has therefore been expressed about the possibility of increasing the odds of developing serotonin syndrome with the combination of 5-HTP and an SSRI drug; however, a recent review on the safety of 5-HTP concludes that 'serotonin syndrome has not been reported in humans in association with 5-HTP, either as monotherapy [on its own] or in combination with other medications'.[134] Another review, published in 2004, concludes that 'no definitive cases of toxicity have emerged despite the worldwide usage of 5-HTP for the last 20 years'.[135]

So, in over 25 years' use there has been no clear case of serotonin syndrome or other significant side effects. Even so, to be on the safe side, I don't recommend you supplement this nutrient, especially in high doses, if you are currently taking SSRI medication.

A small percentage of people, less than 5 per cent, experience nausea on 5-HTP, especially the first time they take it. This is because 5-HTP can be converted into serotonin in the gut, as well as the brain. The serotonin receptors in the gut can overreact if the amount is too high, and nausea can result. If so, just lower the dose. Your body will soon adjust. This effect can be minimised, and the absorption of 5-HTP maximised, by taking your 5-HTP supplement with a carbohydrate food such as an oatcake or a piece of fruit. Otherwise 5-HTP is best absorbed on an empty stomach.

I have heard of a few people who feel more anxious or hyped up on 5-HTP. If you don't feel better on it, it is always possible that you just don't need it. Not everyone has low levels of serotonin. So how do you know?

Are you deficient in serotonin?

It isn't easy to test whether or not you are serotonin deficient, because neither blood nor urine serotonin or tryptophan levels correlate well with the actual level in your brain, or rather the cerebrospinal fluid that your brain swims in. Some labs have measured the breakdown products of serotonin, such as 5HiAA in the urine, but even these tests aren't that good an indicator.

Professor Tapan Audhya, from New York University Medical Center, first showed that the level of serotonin found in platelets – which are tiny disc-like bodies in the blood – correlates with the level of these transmitters in the brain.[136] Next, he investigated whether people with depression do actually have abnormal levels of platelet serotonin by measuring platelet levels in 52 normal and 74 depressed volunteers. The difference was striking. In 73 per cent of depressed patients, serotonin levels were barely a fifth of those in the normal subjects.[137]

Knowing that this neurotransmitter is made directly from amino acids found in food, Audhya then gave his patients 5-HTP. This corrected the deficiency and resulted in major and rapid relief from depression.[138]

When it comes to treating depression or any other chronic condition, nutrition is a real alternative, as it is based on finding out what is actually going on in the patient's system and then sorting out any specific imbalances. That makes a lot more sense, and is far more scientific, than giving millions of people precisely the same chemical regardless of what is actually wrong with them.

At the Brain Bio Centre we test platelet levels of serotonin at Professor Audhya's lab in New York. The trouble is, this test isn't yet widely available. I know of only two laboratories who are offering this test at the moment (see Resources).

CASE STUDY: HOLLY

Holly felt that her anxiety, depression and indecision were ruining her life. She constantly felt stressed, had frequent mood swings, she would cry for no reason and was finding it hard to think straight. When we tested her at the Brain Bio Centre, her serotonin levels were rock bottom. She was also very low in magnesium, which is one of the essential minerals needed to make serotonin, as well as being vital for good sleep. She was recommended a supplement programme to increase her serotonin, including 5-HTP, B vitamins and magnesium. Over the course of her treatment, Holly began to feel much better. She started sleeping well, her anxiety reduced and her mood lifted. Her serotonin level was retested twice, and each time it increased. At her last consultation she was recommended a maintenance supplement programme as she was doing so well. She was amazed at the reduction in anxiety and said it had made a substantial difference and that she felt much more balanced and could see the positive outlook, rather than the negative.

Noradrenalin – the motivation factor

Another neurotransmitter deficiency associated with depression and lack of motivation is adrenalin's 'brother', noradrenalin. That's the 'N' in the new generation of antidepressants, called SNRIs. As you can see in the illustration below, adrenalin and noradrenalin are made from a neurotransmitter called dopamine, which is made from the amino acid tyrosine, which is itself made from the amino acid phenylalanine. Now that we understand the 'family tree' of adrenalin, it is logical to assume

How tyrosine turns into adrenalin and noradrenalin

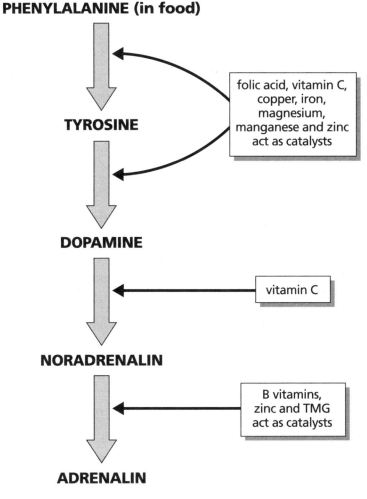

that, if drugs that block the breakdown of these neurotransmitters do elevate mood and motivation, albeit with undesirable side effects, then supplementing the amino acid phenylalanine or tyrosine might work too. And they do, although the evidence, or scale of benefit, isn't nearly as good as for 5-HTP. Let's look at the facts.

The role of tyrosine

In a double-blind study, 150–200mg of the amino acid phenylalanine, or the antidepressant drug imipramine, were administered to 40 depressed patients for one month. Both groups had the same degree of positive results: less depression, anxiety and sleep disturbance.[139] Another group of researchers screened depressed patients by testing phenythylamine in the blood (low levels mean you need more phenylalanine). They then gave 40 depressed patients supplements of phenylalanine, and 31 of them improved.[140]

Tyrosine has been shown to work well in those with dopamine-dependent depression. In a pilot study administering 3,200mg tyrosine a day to 12 patients, a significant improvement in mood and sleep was observed on the very first day.[141]

The military has long known that tyrosine improves mental and physical performance under stress. Recent research from the Netherlands demonstrates how tyrosine gives you the edge in conditions of stress. Twenty-one cadets were put through a demanding one-week military combat training course. Ten cadets were given a drink containing 2g of tyrosine a day, while the remaining 11 were given an identical drink without the tyrosine. Those on tyrosine consistently performed better, both in memorising the task at hand and in tracking the tasks they had performed.[142] Another study found that the normal decline in thinking straight when very cold is mitigated by taking tyrosine. In this case the study participants had less cognitive decline.[143]

However, giving people a tyrosine and phenylalanine-free diet doesn't induce depression in the same way that removing tryptophan can do.[144] This suggests that tyrosine or phenylalanine deficiency is unlikely to be a common cause of depression. So, these amino acids on their own are not as potent as 5-HTP and are more likely to help if you are very stressed, burning the candle at both ends or doing something that really requires endurance. I often supplement tyrosine during a gruelling lecture tour or when I'm climbing mountains.

If you take lots of stimulants, tyrosine may be right for you

Those stimulants and drugs that use up tyrosine and phenylalanine – and are therefore more likely to make you need more – are caffeine, cocaine, speed, tobacco, marijuana, alcohol and sugar. If you are a stimulant junkie, you are more likely to benefit from extra tyrosine. It is also the building block for thyroxine and therefore an essential supplement if you have an underactive thyroid (see Chapter 8).

Testing to find the answers

Of course, the big question is, how do you know what's going to work for you? A more scientific approach would be to check whether depressed patients actually had an imbalance in their neurotransmitters, and if so, exactly which ones were low, so that they could be given a boost. That's what we do at the Brain Bio Centre, but that it is not what happens in general practice. Instead, the diagnosis of depression is based solely on a checklist of psychological symptoms, which doesn't tell you anything about what is going on with brain, or indeed body, chemistry.

When Professor Tapan Audhya tested 52 normal and 74 depressed volunteers, two-thirds of the depressed patients had very low noradrenalin levels and these people did respond to tyrosine supplementation.[145] You are more likely to benefit if you have the following symptoms:

Questionnaire: is your tyrosine depleted?

	Yes	No
1 Do you have a consistently low energy level and little stamina?	☐	☐
2 Do you lack motivation and often feel apathetic?	☐	☐
3 Do you find it hard to concentrate, have poor memory or mental fuzziness?	☐	☐

	Yes	No
4 Do you feel empty or incomplete a lot of the time?	☐	☐
5 Do you find it hard to feel pleasure?	☐	☐
6 Do you tend to overeat or drink alcohol, trying to fill the emptiness you feel?	☐	☐
7 Are you hypersensitive to emotional and physical pain?	☐	☐
8 Do you use or crave stimulants, such as caffeine or nicotine?	☐	☐
9 Are you, or have you been, under a lot of stress?	☐	☐
10 Do you lack sleep?	☐	☐
11 Do you feel physically exhausted?	☐	☐
12 Have you been under a lot of physical stress, including excessive exercise or living in a cold environment?	☐	☐

Score 1 for each 'yes' answer

Total score:

Score

5 or more
There is a good chance that you will benefit from tyrosine supplementation.

How much tyrosine should you take?

If your score suggests that you would benefit from supplementing tyrosine, take 500–1,000mg of tyrosine (or tyrosine plus phenylalanine combined), twice a day, ideally with a carbohydrate snack but away from other protein foods. Start off with the lower dose. Just as for 5-HTP and tryptophan, ensure you have enough catalyst B vitamins. Some supplement combinations provide tyrosine, phenylalanine, 5-HTP and the catalyst B vitamins to hedge your bets.

Essential fats sharpen up your brain's reception or listening skills for neurotransmitters, so make sure you are eating enough fish and/ or taking omega-3-rich fish oil supplements. Also, adrenal hormones are depleted by too much caffeine and sugar. Blood sugar problems lead to too many blood sugar highs and lows, and lows trigger adrenal hormone release. Follow my low-GL mood-boosting diet, explained in Part 3.

If tyrosine is going to help, you should feel the benefits within a week or two. If you don't feel any change within a week, try taking more for three days. If you still feel no different, then it is unlikely that tyrosine deficiency is part of your problem.

Are there any side effects with tyrosine?

Tyrosine supplementation has been tested and may be beneficial for hypertension, stress, cognitive function and memory, addictions, Parkinson's disease, phenylketonuria and narcolepsy, as well as depression. No adverse effects have been reported. (Phenylketonuria is a genetic condition in which a person is unable to convert phenylalanine to tyrosine. Tyrosine is particularly helpful for this condition but phenylalanine must not be given.) However, not that much data is available on long-term toxicity. One area of potential concern relates to people with melanoma. Oxidised tyrosine appears to promote the growth of melanoma cancer cells,[146] so I would not advise tyrosine supplementation if you have melanoma.

Because these are stimulating neurotransmitters, there is a general caution about taking them if you have hypertension (high blood pressure), since adrenalin does raise blood pressure; however, in one study where 2.5g L-tyrosine was given three times daily for two weeks to people with mild essential hypertension, no beneficial or adverse effects were found.[147] If you do have high blood pressure, it is best to monitor this if you are supplementing tyrosine.

Also, if you have difficulty getting to sleep, or find that you become more jittery or 'hyper', stop taking tyrosine or phenylalanine.

Generally, it is better to take tyrosine in the morning, and at noon, than in the evening, because it is a stimulating amino acid.

Foods rich in tyrosine

Individual amino acid supplements are much more potent that just eating foods rich in amino acids, partly because the cocktail of amino acids in foods compete for absorption, and partly because of the amount provided; however, it is always good to make sure your diet provides an optimal amount of tyrosine, or its precursor, phenylalanine. These are found in fish, soy products, poultry, meat, eggs, dairy products, butter beans, almonds, peanuts, sesame seeds, pumpkin seeds, wheatgerm and whole oats. If you are eating foods rich in tryptophan, you are probably also eating foods rich in tyrosine and its precursor l-phenylalanine (see page 108).

We don't just need these amino acids for making noradrenalin, adrenalin and dopamine, which are all motivating neurotransmitters. Phenylalanine is also an essential amino acid for making body proteins such as muscle, and tyrosine is the precursor for the thyroid hormone thyroxine.

SAMe: the master tuner

I have already mentioned SAMe (S-adenosyl methionine) in Part 1 as one of most well-researched natural mood boosters. It sells like hotcakes in the US, and I always stock up when I visit. That's because you can't buy SAMe in Europe, because it's been classified as a 'medicine' and not a food. Over 100 placebo-controlled, double-blind studies show that SAMe is equal, or superior, to antidepressants, and that it works faster, most often within a few days (most pharmaceutical antidepressants may take a few weeks to take effect) and with few side effects. Yet not many doctors ever prescribe it.

Research into SAMe

The following list outlines the results of some of the trials comparing SAMe to conventional antidepressants or placebos.

- In one four-week trial comparing SAMe to a tricyclic antidepressant, 62 per cent of the patients treated with SAMe improved, compared to 50 per cent of those on the drug. Regardless of the type of treatment, patients with a decrease of 50 per cent in their Ham-D score showed a significant increase in plasma SAMe concentration, suggesting that tricyclic drugs may work because they raise SAMe levels.[148]

- Another trial comparing SAMe to the tricyclic drug imipramine found that 67 per cent of the SAMe patients had 50 per cent or greater improvement within two weeks, compared to only 22 per cent on the drug.[149]

- A larger study in Italy confirmed SAMe's fast action in a placebo-controlled, double-blind study.[150] Patients with major depression were given 1,600 mg of SAMe per day. In order to control for the placebo effect, the researchers gave the patients a placebo for a week before beginning the actual trial. Those who improved on the placebo were eliminated from the study. By day ten, SAMe had decreased depression by 27 per cent versus imipramine's 18 per cent on the Ham-D scale.

- In a trial with post-menopausal women, SAMe lowered the depression rating compared to placebo within ten days.[151] Other studies have confirmed that SAMe is a highly effective antidepressant with a fraction of the side effects.[152]

- According to one comprehensive review of all the studies, 92 per cent of those with depression responded to SAMe, compared to 85 per cent for the medications.[153]

Is SAMe safe?

SAMe is a safe, natural amino acid, normally made from the essential amino acid methionine. No toxicity has been reported, even at much higher doses than the therapeutic amounts of 800–1,600mg daily. Occasionally, some people experience mild to moderate nausea, heartburn or stomach ache when starting on 800mg twice daily on an empty stomach mid morning and mid afternoon. Therefore, it is best to start with 200mg twice a day for several days and then to slowly increase to 800mg twice a day. It is best absorbed on an empty stomach.

In general, side effects in SAMe studies are few and mild. In some studies, SAMe caused fewer or less serious side effects than the placebo! In a double-blind study with 734 people comparing SAMe with the painkiller drug Naproxen or a placebo, 10 people withdrew from the study due to side effects from SAMe, compared to 13 from the placebo and 17 from Naproxen.[154]

The most commonly reported side effects are gastrointestinal – primarily heartburn, nausea and stomach ache. There have been occasional reports of mania (excessive mood elevation and overstimulation), but this side effect is much rarer; however, for this reason, people with bipolar disorder who wish to take SAMe must do so with caution, and only under the supervision of a doctor.

SAMe has side benefits, however, including being an effective treatment for degenerative joint disease, fibromyalgia and liver problems.

How to take SAMe

You need 400–1,600mg a day, but the trouble is it's been classified as a medicine in the EU, which effectively means it's no longer available in health-food stores. In the UK you can, however, obtain it on prescription from your doctor. You can get it in other countries, or via the Internet for your own use. SAMe is quite expensive and not very stable, so make sure you get it in the form of butanedisulfonate, which is more stable. Keep it refrigerated. Another form that I like is S-adenosyl-L-methionine tosylate disulfate that comes in sealed 'blister packs' to protect against oxidation and which doesn't need refrigeration.

Generally, it is best to start with 200mg twice a day for several days and then to slowly increase up to 800mg twice a day. The protective blister packs should not be opened before you are ready to take the supplements, and the tablet should not be cut in half to achieve a lower dose, because the SAMe may break down or oxidise before you have taken the second half. It should be taken on an empty stomach for the best absorption.

An alternative that is much more stable and less costly is TMG (tri-methyl-glycine). In the body it turns into SAMe, but you need to supplement three times as much. Try supplementing 600–2,000mg a day, again on an empty stomach or with fruit. Start with the lower dose. (I'll explain more about TMG in Chapter 13 when we explore the vital importance of methylation nutrients and how they make you feel more connected.) Together with B_6, B_{12} and folic acid, your body can then make its own SAMe. In truth, there isn't anything like the same level of research for TMG, but the body can easily convert it into SAMe.

It's SAMe that improves communication between cells – something that I'll be explaining in detail in Chapter 13 on methylation. SAMe acts as a natural stimulant and motivator, helping to keep you on an 'up'. Most people experience these benefits within days of supplementing SAMe. So, taking SAMe is a bit like fuel-injecting your car. It really does give a very effective mood boost when you need it.

Eat the best foods

As well as supplementing SAMe, or TMG plus B vitamins, it's a good idea to eat foods rich in it. As you'll see in Chapter 13, when we start to explore the vital role of methylating nutrients, TMG is rich in methyl groups that help your brain to stay in tune. So too are foods rich in choline, which turns into TMG. Eggs and organ meats are by far the best food sources of choline, whereas nuts, seeds, beans and root vegetables are rich sources of TMG. TMG is also concentrated in the bran and the germ of grains, so it is important to eat whole grains.[155] Lecithin or lecithin granules, which you can buy in a health-food store, are a vegetarian source of choline. SAMe itself is made from an essential amino acid, methionine, which is found in all protein foods.

SUMMARY

- If you score high on the serotonin check (page 104), add 100mg of 5-HTP to your daily supplement programme. You need a basic intake of B vitamins – B_6, B_{12} and folic acid, plus niacin (B_3) – as well as zinc and magnesium to maximise the conversion of 5-HTP to serotonin, but these will be provided by your basic high-potency multivitamin–mineral. Take 5-HTP with a carbohydrate snack, such as some fruit, away from meals, or 15 minutes before a meal. You can take twice this amount, 200mg a day, morning and afternoon, but don't take 5-HTP if you are on antidepressant drugs.

- If you scored high on the tyrosine check on page 117 you should also take 500–1,000mg of tyrosine. L-tyrosine, the

CONTINUED...

natural form of this amino acid, is available in supplements of 500mg. I recommend supplementing 500mg twice a day, morning and afternoon, ideally away from, or before, a main meal, with a carbohydrate snack. Some formulas provide both 5-HTP and tyrosine.

- If you live in a country where you can buy SAMe, try taking 400mg a day (200mg twice a day on an empty stomach) for a couple of days, then increase the dose to 400mg twice a day. If you experience any nausea or stomach ache, lower the dose. Consult your doctor before taking SAMe if you are prone to manic states or phases.
- See Part 3 for your complete Mood-boosting Action Plan.

Chapter 12

THE IMPORTANCE OF A GOOD NIGHT'S SLEEP

There's a big link between how much and how well you sleep and how you feel the next day. Obviously, if you don't sleep enough and feel tired the next day that doesn't put you in a good mood, but as this chapter will show, there's more to it than that. More than a quarter of those who are frequently sleep deficient report low mood symptoms.[156] In our 100% Health Survey of 55,570 people, more than half (55 per cent) reported difficulty sleeping or restless sleep, whereas more, almost two-thirds (63 per cent), felt like they needed more sleep.

To help identify if you are suffering from excessive daytime sleepiness and poor quality of sleep, complete the questionnaire below, which uses the Epworth Sleepiness Scale, a well-proven way of finding out if you are getting enough.

Questionnaire: check for excessive daytime sleepiness (the Epworth Sleepiness Scale)

Rate the chance that you would doze off or fall asleep during the following daytime situations from 0 to 3, as below:

0 means you would never doze off or fall asleep in a given situation.
1 means there is a slight chance that you would doze off or fall asleep.
2 means there is a moderate chance that you would doze off or fall asleep.
3 means there is a high chance that you would doze off or fall asleep.

Situation

1 Sitting and reading. ☐

2 Sitting inactive in a public place (such as a theatre, lecture or meeting). ☐

3 Watching TV. ☐

4 As a passenger in a car for an hour or longer without a break. ☐

5 Lying down to rest in the afternoon. ☐

6 Sitting and talking to someone. ☐

7 In a car, while stopped in traffic. ☐

Total score: ☐

Score

10 or more

You most likely suffer from excessive daytime sleepiness, a strong indication that you are sleep deprived and need to improve the quality and/or duration of your sleep. People who continue to suffer from poor sleep are more prone to depression, anxiety, drug cravings and relapse.

Improving your quantity and quality of sleep

So, how do you get sufficient quantity and a good quality of sleep? Obviously, stress and worries can be a contributor to poor sleep, but understanding the biochemistry of sleep, and what you can do to tilt the odds in your favour, can even help reduce your stress levels and get you out of the vicious cycle whereby a lack of sleep keeps making you more stressed and depressed. Biochemically speaking, mood and sleep have a lot in common. The amino acid 5-HTP, which we discussed in Chapter 11, is not only the raw material for serotonin, but also for melatonin, which helps you sleep, controlling the sleep–wake cycle. It's the brain's neurotransmitter that keeps you in sync with the earth's day–night cycle. Jet lag, for example, happens when the brain's chemistry takes time to catch up with a sudden time-zone shift. What's happening inside your brain is that melatonin, which should be released at night so that you sleep, is released in the 'old' night-time. Taking melatonin just before bed in the new time zone helps to reset your brain's chemistry to recover from jet lag.

How the brain makes melatonin

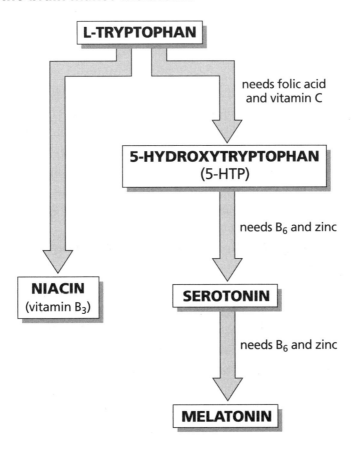

Melatonin: the sleep hormone

As you start to wind down in the evening, serotonin levels rise and adrenalin levels fall. As it gets darker, melatonin kicks in. Melatonin is an almost identical molecule to serotonin, from which it is made, and both are made from 5-HTP, itself derived from the amino acid tryptophan, which is present in most protein foods.

One way to improve matters is to provide more of the building blocks that are used to make serotonin and that means 5-HTP (5-hydroxytryptophan), which in turn is made from tryptophan – a conversion process that requires folic acid, vitamin B_6, vitamin C and zinc. So you've got a biochemical chain stretching straight from foods that are particularly high in tryptophan – like chicken, cheese, tuna, tofu, eggs, nuts, seeds and milk – up to melatonin. Other foods associated with inducing sleep are lettuce and oats. To support your brain's ability to turn tryptophan into serotonin and melatonin, it's best to supplement a high-potency multivitamin that contains at least 200mcg of folic acid, 20mg of vitamin B_6, 10mg of zinc and 100mg of vitamin C.

Alternatively, you could supplement these natural chemicals directly. Melatonin, which is a neurotransmitter, not a nutrient, is proven to help you get to sleep, but it needs to be used much more cautiously than a nutrient. In controlled trials, it's about a third as effective as the commonly prescribed sleeping pills, but has a fraction of the side effects.[157] If you have difficulty getting to sleep, perhaps only going to sleep very late, and you are prone to feeling low, it's particularly effective both for helping you sleep and for improving your mood.[158]

Even so, supplementing too much can have undesirable effects, such as diarrhoea, constipation, nausea, dizziness, reduced libido, headaches, depression and nightmares; so, if you do suffer from the above problems you may want to try between 3mg and 6mg before bedtime. In Britain, melatonin is classified as a medicine and is only available on prescription. Discuss this option with your doctor. It is available over the counter in other countries, such as the US and South Africa, and on the Internet from those countries. I don't recommend melatonin on a long-term basis, but it can be very useful to bring you back into balance.

Help from 5-HTP and tryptophan

Another option is to take 5-HTP (see Chapter 11). Supplementing 100–200mg one hour before you go to bed helps you to get a good night's sleep.[159] It's also been shown to reduce sleep terrors in children when given at an amount equivalent to 1mg per pound of bodyweight before bed.[160] 5-HTP is best taken on an empty stomach, or with a small amount of carbohydrate, such as an oatcake or a piece of fruit, one hour before sleep.

Tryptophan has also proven consistently effective in promoting sleep, if taken in amounts ranging from 1–4g.[161] Smaller doses have not proven effective. You also need to take it at least 45 minutes before you want to go to sleep, again ideally with a small amount of carbohydrate, such as an oatcake. The reason for this is that eating carbohydrate causes a release of insulin, and insulin carries tryptophan into the brain.

Sometimes supplementing tryptophan, 5-HTP or melatonin for a month can bring you back into balance, re-establishing proper sleep patterns. Doing this will make it much easier for you to wean yourself off the more harmful sleeping pills, if you are taking them. Once you're off the sleeping pills, continue with melatonin or 5-HTP for a month, then switch from melatonin to 5-HTP for a month or continue taking 5-HTP, then try stopping this as well. By this time your brain chemistry should be back in balance and you may find that you sleep just fine.

What about any side effects?

Tryptophan can make you drowsy if you take it during the daytime. And there's one important caution. If you are on SSRI antidepressants, which block the recycling of serotonin, and you also take large amounts of 5-HTP, this could theoretically make too much serotonin. An excess of serotonin can be as risky as too little (see page 112). Although this hasn't been reported, I don't recommend combining the two.

Switching off the adrenalin will also help you sleep

Although you need adequate serotonin and melatonin to give you a good night's sleep, anything that helps you switch off adrenalin in the evening will help you get to sleep more easily. In fact, there's a big link between feeling emotionally reactive, not sleeping well and consequently being prone to feeling low.[162]

So, how do you switch off adrenalin, relax and get a good night's sleep, and consequently feel better in the morning? Avoiding caffeine, at least after midday, is a no-brainer, because caffeine suppresses melatonin for up to ten hours.[163] I recommend none after midday, and that includes green tea, if you have difficulty getting to sleep.

The main neurotransmitter that switches off adrenalin is called GABA (gamma-amino-butyric acid). This is both an amino acid and a neurotransmitter. In the US and some other countries you can buy it over the counter in health-food stores and pharmacies. In the EU it is classified as a medicine and is therefore available only on prescription. This is a real shame, because GABA is a natural antidote to anxiety and the inability to relax. Almost all sleeping pills and anti-anxiety drugs work to promote a GABA-like effect. The trouble with these is that they either interfere with your body's own ability to make GABA or make you less responsive to it. The net result is that when you try to get off these drugs you are likely to develop extreme anxiety and insomnia. My book *How to Quit Without Feeling S**t* explains how to come off these drugs, which needs to be done with professional guidance and support.

Many people use alcohol to relax. This promotes GABA, switching off adrenalin, but it only works for an hour or so. When the effects wear off, you want another drink. If you go to sleep under the influence of alcohol, it disturbs the normal sleep cycle, which can promote low moods. The net consequence of regular alcohol consumption is GABA depletion, which leads to more adrenalin, anxiety and emotional oversensitivity and less good-quality sleep.

How much GABA should you take?

In the US and other countries you can buy GABA in 500mg capsules. Taking one to three an hour before bed helps promote a good night's sleep. The combination of GABA and 5-HTP is even better. In a placebo-controlled trial this combination cut time taken to fall asleep from 32 minutes to 19 minutes and extended sleep from five to almost seven hours.[164] Taking 1,000mg of GABA, plus 100mg of 5-HTP is a recipe for a good night's sleep.

Nutrients and herbs for sleep

If you have trouble sleeping supplement 100mg of 5-HTP and, if you live in a country where you can buy it, 1,000mg of GABA an hour before bed. If you can't get GABA, taurine and glutamine are precursors. Some formulas provide these in combination with calming herbs such as hops and passionflower. Valerian is classified as a 'medicinal herb', being more potent, and is not included in such formulas. It's a good alternative to GABA, if you just can't get to sleep and you live in a country that prohibits GABA – such as in the EU – but don't take both.

Some formulas containing 5-HTP and herbs also include magnesium, which calms the nervous system and has been reported to help reduce restless legs and insomnia.[165] Deficiency is certainly a potential reason for feeling low or anxious. I supplement 200mg every day and recommend 300mg if you are feeling low. Combinations of these various elements are particularly effective (see Resources).

Valerian is the most potent GABA-promoting herb and, as such, can also promote daytime drowsiness, so it's best to take it only in the evening if you have anxiety or insomnia and an inability to 'switch off'. Valerian is sometimes referred to as 'nature's Valium'. As such, it can interact with alcohol and other sedative drugs and should therefore be taken in combination with them only under careful medical supervision. It seems to work in two ways: by promoting the body's release of GABA and by providing the amino acid glutamine, from which the brain can make GABA. Neither of these mechanisms makes it addictive.[166] One double-blind study in which participants took 60mg of valerian 30 minutes before bedtime for 28 days found it to be as effective as oxazepam, a drug used to treat anxiety.[167] Another found it to be highly effective in reducing insomnia compared with placebos.[168] A review of studies to date cites six studies that show a significant benefit.[169] My experience is that it works exceptionally well for many people. To help you sleep, take 150–300mg about 45 minutes before bedtime.

Music to switch off your brain

New York psychiatrist Dr Galina Mindlin, uses 'brain music' – rhythmic patterns of sounds derived from recordings of patients' own brainwaves

– to help them overcome insomnia, anxiety and depression. A small double-blind study from 1998, conducted at Toronto University in Canada, found that 80 per cent of those undergoing this treatment reported benefits.[170]

Another study found that specially composed music induced a shift in brainwave patterns to alpha waves, associated with the deep relaxation you experience before you go to sleep. In a study of patients going to the dentist, this was found to induce less anxiety.[171] This music, composed by John Levine to induce a relaxation response, sounds like very calming classical piano music. It is designed to switch the brainwaves from beta waves, associated with adrenalin and excitation, to alpha waves, which is a prerequisite for going to sleep. My favourite CD is called *Silence of Peace* (see Resources), and I receive many testimonials from people who have found almost immediate relief from insomnia by listening to it.

CASE STUDY: SUE

Sue had been suffering from post traumatic stress disorder, sleeping for about three hours, then waking every 45 minutes or so. Here's what she says:

'I ordered, almost wearily, the Orange Grove Siesta *CD for insomnia and* Silence of Peace. *They came the next day and I duly dusted off my Walkman to use with the CDs in bed. The improvement happened from night one; now, just one week later, I am sleeping for six to seven hours. If I wake, which is becoming rare, I simply tune in again! I haven't heard the end of the CD yet.'*

Psychological approaches

Having a lot of stress and things on your mind is a major factor causing insomnia and low mood, but seeing a psychotherapist is likely to help. A small study published in a 2004 issue of the *Archives of Internal Medicine* found that just two hours of cognitive behavioural therapy (CBT) was able to cure insomnia by encouraging patients to acknowledge the stress that was preventing them from sleeping and then helping them develop ways of dealing with it.[172] One way CBT works is by helping the patient identify negative or unhelpful thoughts – such as, 'I just can't sleep without my pills' – and then encouraging them to challenge them – such as, 'I didn't have a problem until six months ago', or 'I fell asleep with no trouble after that long walk.'

Such techniques are often combined with progressive muscle relaxation, or a form of biofeedback to reduce the amount of active beta brainwaves before going to bed. This involves hooking a patient up to a machine that displays their brainwaves on a screen. They can then see the brainwaves slowing down as they practise relaxation techniques such as slowing their breathing. The basic principle of biofeedback is becoming aware of a biological function, such as your heart rate or breathing, and by focusing on this it naturally slows down. In a way, this is the dynamics of basic meditation: by focusing on the breath, your breathing naturally slows down and becomes more relaxed.

A very effective technique is called Heart Math. (See Resources to find a Heart Math practitioner.)

SLEEP HYGIENE: MAKING THE BEST ENVIRONMENT FOR GOOD SLEEP

This piece of advice forms part of most sleep regimes. Keep the bedroom quiet, dark and at a temperature that's appropriate for you. Wear comfortable clothing. Don't have a big meal in the evening, and avoid coffee and alcohol at least three hours before you go to bed. Also, exercise regularly but not within three hours of bedtime. Be aware that certain prescription medications can cause insomnia, such as steroids, bronchodilators (used for asthma) and diuretics.

Good habits

The idea of 'sleep hygiene' is to create regular sleep-promoting habits. A similar but more systematic approach is known as 'stimulus control therapy' (SCT). This involves ensuring that the bed is only associated with sleeping. Patients are advised against having naps, and to go to bed when sleepy, to get up within 20 minutes if they haven't fallen asleep, to do something relaxing until they feel drowsy and to try again – but to get up again if it fails.

Although sleep hygiene is widely recommended, there have been very few studies of it as an individual treatment, and those found a 'limited improvement'. The evidence for the effectiveness of SCT is much stronger. Regular exercise also helps, as I'll show you in Chapter 14. Ask your doctor about getting psychological help, or contact the Sleep Assessment Advisory Service (see Resources). Also, in the Resources section I list other psychotherapy organisations.

The secret of dreaming

Your dreams are the way your brain frees your mind of the emotions of the day. Your brain continues to work through problems during your dream-state, so that you can wake up feeling refreshed. Bad sleep, with no dreams, denies your brain of this important function, causing you to feel low; but if you have too many unresolved worries, these will overload and disrupt your sleep, also resulting in low moods.

After a couple of hours' sleep, we enter the dream-state sleep, known as rapid eye movement, or REM, stage 1. REM sleep normally occurs 90 minutes after the onset of sleep, but if we are sleep-deprived it may occur within 30 minutes.

Dreaming occurs during REM sleep and most of us have four or more REM periods per night, even though many people have difficulty remembering the dreams that occur in them. As well as providing physical rest, sleep may provide the chance to make a 'back-up tape' of the day's events for our large 'computer': the brain. Although Westerners pay little heed to dreams, one African tribe believe that 'real life' is lived in dreams and that daytime is the illusion. The Bolivian philosopher Oscar Ichazo describes dream reality like the stars at night: that dream thoughts are always happening, but the brightness of the sun, daytime consciousness, blots them out.

Nutrition to aid dream sleep

Many scientists believe that nutritional deficiency is one reason why poor or no dream recall occurs. In a survey at the ION we found that more than 40 per cent of people had no, or very infrequent, dream recall. When researching the signs and symptoms of vitamin B_6 and zinc deficiency, we found that an alarming proportion of deficient people couldn't recall their dreams. After supplementing with vitamin B_6 and zinc, their dream recall returned and they reported their dreams as being more vivid. If you don't dream, try supplementing up to 200mg of vitamin B_6 and 20mg of zinc, starting with half this amount. If this doesn't have an effect within three days, take the full amount. I have certainly had many clients report that they start dreaming, or remembering their dreams, on a regular basis once they change their diet and take nutritional supplements.

Working through problems in our sleep

Psychologists Joe Griffin and Ivan Tyrrell have made extensive investigations into how dreaming allows you to discharge unexpressed emotions during the day, and why depressed people so often wake up exhausted and without motivation. They describe in their book, *How to Lift Depression*, how emotions we couldn't express and complete at the time become expressed in dreams. Try this simple exercise:

If you have a dream in which the predominant emotion is that you are angry or frightened, for example, scan the day before for moments when you experienced that feeling and were unable to express how you felt.

We dream to deactivate unexpressed emotions. Griffin and Tyrell find that many people with a tendency to depression are reacting emotionally on a much more frequent basis – worrying, getting anxious, feeling grumpy, getting upset – and have more undischarged emotional content in the day. At night, they have more REM dreaming, which is itself exhausting, because they spend less time in the deeper, recuperative sleep. Also, the authors propose that we only have so much motivational energy, so if you have an overactive dream process, in which you are over-aroused, the net effect is that when you wake up, your get up and go has got up and gone!

Based on this theory, Griffin and Tyrell have developed psychotherapeutic techniques, which are part of a new school of psychology called the Human Givens Approach, aimed at helping people deal with depression. Many psychotherapists train in these techniques, and the book itself takes you through some very helpful exercises. There is also a one-day workshop you can go on. You may find the exercises help you, especially if you are waking up tired, exhausted and depressed. To find out more go to Resources.

SUMMARY

- Find the right kind of psychotherapy; cognitive behavioural therapy is especially recommended.
- Practise 'sleep hygiene'.
- Exercise regularly but not within a few hours of sleep.
- Listen to alpha-wave-inducing music while in bed, and practise relaxation techniques.
- Eat more green leafy vegetables, nuts and seeds to ensure you're getting enough magnesium, and consider supplementing 300mg of magnesium in the evening with or without calcium (500mg).
- Supplement 100mg of 5-HTP and – if you live in a country where you can buy it – take 1,000mg of GABA an hour before bed. If you can't get GABA, taurine and glutamine are precursors. Some formulas provide this in combination with calming herbs.
- Consider taking valerian, hops, passionflower, St John's wort or a 'sleep formula' combining several of them. Choose a standardised extract or tincture, and follow the dosage instructions.
- Avoid sugar and caffeine, and minimise your intake of alcohol. Don't combine alcohol with sleeping pills or anti-anxiety medication.
- If you feel the need for a sleeping pill, ask your doctor to prescribe melatonin, in which case don't take extra 5-HTP.
- See Part 3 for your complete Mood-boosting Action Plan.

Chapter 13

GET YOURSELF CONNECTED WITH UPLIFTING B VITAMINS

One of the most important processes in the brain and body is called methylation, which is totally dependent on your intake of specific B vitamins. In this chapter I'll be explaining how poor methylation affects your mood and how you can improve it by taking the appropriate nutrients.

The process of methylation is how your body keeps thousands of neurotransmitters, hormones and other essential biochemicals in balance. This is quite a feat; there are something like a million methylation reactions every second. So your methylation ability is a critical factor in determining your mood, motivation, concentration and ability to deal with stress. Here's an example: if the fire alarm goes off at work, you'll be pumping adrenalin in 0.2 seconds – ready to act, literally, in a split second – but none of this would happen without methylation, as it's this process that manufactures the adrenalin.

To get a bit technical, the manufacturing process hinges on a small unit of organic compounds, which is known as a 'methyl group'. The adrenalin is made when one of these methyl groups is added by the amino acid SAMe (the hero in Chapter 11) to noradrenalin. Methylation also helps to make the brain-friendly fats called phospholipids (see page 91) and even controls gene expression, which is how the information in a gene is translated into action, affecting how you think and feel. Exactly how all this works is explained on page 142.

Methylation is linked to a number of mental states and conditions. Faulty methylation is now known to predict depression, affect concentration and the ability to stay in touch with reality. So, ascertaining your 'methyl IQ' is important. Luckily, it's easily done by measuring the level of homocysteine – a toxic amino acid – in the blood. I call this the H factor.

The H factor: how this affects your mood

The higher your homocysteine level, the more likely you are to feel low and de-motivated. Many different research groups have proven this association.[173] The ideal is 7 or lower. If you have a high level, above 15, you double your chances of being depressed; for example, a study of women who were tested for homocysteine levels in the blood found that a high level doubled the likelihood of depression.[174] In another study, more than half of those with severe depression were found to have high homocysteine levels.[175]

One of the main reasons for having a high homocysteine level is that you are not receiving sufficient B vitamins, but how much you need partly depends on the genes you inherit. Most important are vitamins B_6, B_{12} and folic acid or folate. Low levels of these are also an excellent predictor of low mood; for example, a recent study reports that men with the highest blood levels of folic acid – that's the B vitamin found in greens and beans – have half the risk of depression.[176] Many other studies have shown the same thing, says a review by scientists at the University of York and Hull York Medical School of 11 studies involving 15,315 people. The review concluded that the lower a person's folate levels the greater is their risk of depression.[177] Having a low level of folate and B_{12} and a high homocysteine level puts you at high risk of depression.[178] Having a low level of B_6 does too.[179] And the higher your B_{12} level the more likely you are to feel better faster.[180] Among older people, giving supplements improves mood.[181]

Mood-lowering folic acid

More importantly, lowering your homocysteine level and increasing your intake of critical nutrients, such as folic acid, improves mood.[182] Overall, for every five depressed people given folic acid, one will experience a 50 per cent drop on the Ham-D scale as a result. So the odds of it helping are about one in five. In one study, depressed people were either given an SSRI antidepressant with folic acid or the SSRI with a placebo. Ninety-three per cent of women taking the SSRI with folic acid had a greater than 50 per cent drop on their Ham-D score, compared to 63 per cent taking the SSRI with placebo.[183] In this study men didn't seem to benefit. Also, the women's homocysteine levels reduced significantly, but the men's didn't, suggesting that you are only likely to get an effect if your homocysteine level comes down.

Testing for homocysteine

Ideally, your homocysteine level should be no higher than 7. It's easily measured by your doctor, or you can do it yourself using a home test kit that you send off to a lab (see Resources). If you live in Germany, having your homocysteine level measured will be routine medical practice. They run millions of tests a year. In the UK, however, getting your level tested, especially for depression, is almost unheard of. At the Brain Bio Centre we always measure homocysteine levels because we have found it to be such an important factor in mood and general mental health.

CASE STUDY: AMANDA-JANE

> Amanda-Jane, aged 33, was suffering with chronic fatigue and low mood, so she decided to check her homocysteine level. She was shocked when she found her H score was 25.9 units. She followed my homocysteine-lowering diet and took a combination of methylation supplements. Almost immediately her sleep improved, and within four weeks she had much more energy. Two months later she re-tested her homocysteine level and found it had dropped to 9.4 units. That's a 64 per cent decrease. Here's what she told me:
>
> *'I feel much better. I'm very busy right now, and in the past I'd feel overwhelmed and not able to cope, both mentally and physically, but now I feel great. My mood is very positive – no panic or depression. I feel buoyant, energetic and enthusiastic. I haven't had any colds or infections. I'm sleeping much better and my PMS has disappeared – I experienced no breast tenderness, mood swings or*

tearfulness during my last period. I am really delighted and will continue the H Factor approach, not quite so strictly, but at a level that I can easily maintain for life.'

Adjusting the level for your age

Your homocysteine level does tend to go up with age and the absolute best level to have if you are over 40 is not much more than your age divided by 10. So if you are 70, a homocysteine level of not more than 8 is good. If you are 40, the ideal would be below 5.

The older you are the less able you are to absorb vitamin B_{12}. A study showed that two people in five over the age of 61 are B_{12} deficient, causing the brain size to shrink; the more deficient they were the more the brain shrank.[184] A Chinese study of 669 people aged over 55 concluded that having a low B_{12} level more than doubles your odds of feeling depressed, and also found that high homocysteine and low folate levels accurately predicts depression.[185]

Are you genetically programmed for low moods?

Some people are much more prone to high homocysteine levels and low moods, and consequently need more B vitamins. This is largely to do with the genes that they inherit. If you look at the illustration on page 143, all the boxed initials are enzymes that drive a key step in the methylation process. These enzymes can be 'up-regulated', meaning they work harder than they should, or 'down-regulated', meaning they are sluggish, or just right. Some of us inherit versions of specific genes that provide the instructions to make these enzymes that work too hard or are sluggish. These differences are called 'gene polymorphisms', much like having blonde or brown hair. Each one of these variations has a particular code name; for example, a polymorphism of the MTHFR gene, which makes the MTHFR enzyme – the enzyme that helps your body to make it's own SAMe, boosting your mood – is called C677TT. Roughly one in ten people have C677TT, which ultimately lessens their ability to create SAMe, the amino acid that's the most important methyl donor in the body.

Supplementing a particular form of B_{12}, 'methyl' B_{12}, or 'methyl' folate or tri-methyl-glycine (TMG) also helps. Approximately one in three of us inherit a variation of one or more of these key genes that makes these key enzymes, MTHFR just being one of them. In one landmark study from the University of California, giving extra B vitamins 'corrected' the deficiency in four out of five inherited 'negative' variations.[186]

You can actually test for all these gene variations (see tests in Resources), which might tell you that you are more likely to need more of specific B vitamins. Your need for B vitamins, however, actually depends both on genes and your diet and lifestyle (for example, coffee raises homocysteine, thus increasing your need for B vitamins, and so does excessive exercise), so it's better to cut to the chase and know your homocysteine level.

How much should you take?

Although there are RDAs (recommended daily allowances) for nutrients, we are all different, and these levels don't take into account genetic individuality. They are therefore only useful as a basic guideline to make sure that you are not going to develop scurvy if you only eat cornflakes, for example, but are not as useful as a guide to what you need to stay healthy and happy.

So, how do you know what you need in the way of folic acid, B_{12}, B_6 and zinc? You can test for each one, but if you don't have enough of any of them, your homocysteine level is going to be high. So the best single indicator is to check your homocysteine level. If it's high, then you know you need more of one or several of these nutrients.

CASE STUDY: CHRIS

Chris felt very unwell, with constant tiredness, worsening memory and concentration, and little zest for life, even though he had no diagnosed disease as such. He felt depressed and brain dead, with no sex drive. When tested, his homocysteine score was 119! That kind of level only really happens if you've inherited one of the defective genes I have been describing and you lack B vitamins.

He followed my recommendations, including high doses

of all these methylation nutrients, for three months. His homocysteine level dropped to 19. After six months it dropped to 11. After a year it was 9. He cannot believe how well he feels. His mood, memory and concentration are completely restored, his energy is so good he now exercises for an hour every day, and his sex drive has returned. He said:

'You have saved my life, or at least made it worth living again.'

HOW NUTRIENTS IMPROVE METHYLATION AND LOWER HOMOCYSTEINE

Looking at the illustration opposite, you will see that the starting point is 'food protein'. The goal is to be able to carry out methylation processes, shown by the arrows on the right-hand side. Food protein contains the amino acid methionine, which then becomes homocysteine. It is then turned, step-by-step, into SAMe by a process that involves a number of enzymes (shown in white boxes). These enzymes are dependent on nutrients (shown in grey boxes). Provided you have enough of these nutrients, the enzymes help to liberate the methyl groups (shown as dots [.]). The cycle on the left liberates a methyl group from folate to help turn homocysteine into SAMe in the cycle on the right. This requires enough B_{12} and folate, primarily, but also B_2 and B_3 (niacin).

Another way to turn homocysteine into SAMe involves the BHMT enzyme, which is dependent on the nutrient TMG, plus zinc. (Although it isn't shown in this diagram, there's another pathway that shunts homocysteine to SAMe that depends on vitamin B_6, zinc and magnesium.)

The goal is to make enough SAMe, which then 'donates' these methyl groups, shown as dots, to keep your brain and body chemistry in balance. It then turns back into homocysteine and can be 'reloaded' back to SAMe provided you have enough of these nutrients. So the critical 'methylation' nutrients are:

Vitamin B_2	Vitamin B_{12}	TMG
Vitamin B_6	Folic acid	Zinc
Magnesium		

The methylation cycle

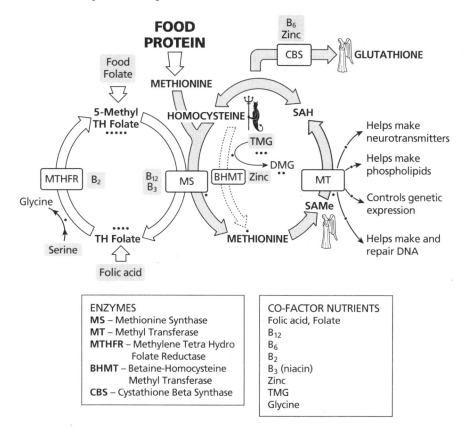

ENZYMES
MS – Methionine Synthase
MT – Methyl Transferase
MTHFR – Methylene Tetra Hydro
Folate Reductase
BHMT – Betaine-Homocysteine
Methyl Transferase
CBS – Cystathione Beta Synthase

CO-FACTOR NUTRIENTS
Folic acid, Folate
B_{12}
B_6
B_2
B_3 (niacin)
Zinc
TMG
Glycine

You can see this methyl cycle as an animated film at www.patrickholford.com/methylation

Do you need to supplement methylation nutrients?

Although there is merit in everyone having a high-potency multivitamin and mineral supplement providing the key methylation nutrients, whether or not you need larger amounts depends on your homocysteine level; however, whether you are likely to benefit from larger amounts also depends very much on whether you have high homocysteine or low B vitamin status. If you don't have the means to get tested, but you score high on the methyl check below, then you are more likely to benefit from larger intakes of methylation nutrients.

Questionnaire: check your methyl IQ

	Yes	No
1 Are you tired a lot of the time?	☐	☐
2 Is your stamina, or ability to keep going, noticeably decreasing?	☐	☐
3 Are you having a hard time keeping your weight stable?	☐	☐
4 Do you often experience physical pain, be it arthritis, muscle aches or migraines?	☐	☐
5 Have you ever suffered from cardiovascular problems or high blood pressure?	☐	☐
6 Do you easily become angry?	☐	☐
7 Do you have difficulty concentrating or easily become confused?	☐	☐
8 Is your mental clarity or concentration decreasing?	☐	☐
9 Are you experiencing more sleeping problems?	☐	☐
10 Is your memory on the decline?	☐	☐
11 Are you often depressed?	☐	☐
12 Do you average two or more alcoholic beverages daily?	☐	☐
13 Do you drink coffee daily?	☐	☐
	Yes	No
14 Do you smoke cigarettes daily?	☐	☐
15 Are you a strict vegan?	☐	☐
16 Do you rarely eat beans, lentils, nuts or seeds?	☐	☐
17 Do you often have less than one serving of green leafy vegetables a day?	☐	☐

Score 1 for each 'yes' answer

Total score:

Score

0–2

Well done! Although the ideal score is of course '0', you do not appear to be experiencing significant problems connected with poor methylation.

3–4

You are beginning to show signs of reduced 'methyl IQ'. Identify your key areas and focus on improving these. By cleaning up your diet and following the advice in Part 3, you'll soon start to see improvements.

5–7

There is a possibility that your homocysteine level is raised, and I suggest you test it. By following the advice in this chapter, together with the dietary and supplement programme in Part 3, you will probably soon start to see an improvement in your symptoms.

Overleaf, you'll see the level of nutrients we give a person at the Brain Bio Centre, depending on their homocysteine level. In the column that relates to a homocysteine level of 6 or less are levels that a good multivitamin and mineral supplement programme would give you. I take these every day and recommend you do the same. But if your homocysteine level is 11, for example, which is probably close to the national average, I'd be recommending much higher nutrient levels. I'd recommend 500mcg of B_{12}, not just 10mcg.

Now, the RDA for B_{12}, which is only found in food of animal origin such as meat, fish, eggs and milk, is only 1mcg in the EU and 2.5mcg in the USA! You could conceivably eat 5mcg but never 500mcg. Why so high? The answer is that only this kind of level of B_{12} corrects mild deficiency – that's what the research shows. To quote one such trial, 'The lowest dose of oral B_{12} required to normalize mild B_{12} deficiency is more than 250 times greater than the RDA, (2.5mcg).'[187] The reason you need so much more B_{12} if you are deficient is because it is hard to absorb, especially as you get older, and you need to take in a lot more orally to get a little more into the blood. That's why some people have B_{12} shots instead, often reporting an uplifted mood after receiving them.

Supplemental B vitamins depending on your H score

Nutrient	No risk below 6	Low risk 6–8	High risk 9–14	Very high risk above 15
Folic acid	200mcg	400mcg	800mcg	1,000mcg
Methyl-B_{12}	10mcg	250mcg	500mcg	1,000mcg
B_6	25mg	50mg	75mg	100mg
B_2	10mg	15mg	20mg	50mg
Zinc	5mg	10mg	15mg	20mg
TMG	500mg	750mg	1–1.5g	3–6g

The good news is that there are supplements that provide all these methylation nutrients in a single pill (see Resources). If your level is high, or very high, you may need to take two or three a day. Have a look at the doses and the instructions on the packet. Also, some homocysteine test results explain what to take.

Monitor your supplementation

Do bear in mind that this combination of nutrients is so effective at lowering your homocysteine level that you don't need to take this quantity for very long. In fact, a very high level of folic acid can be detrimental. So I advise you to re-test your homocysteine level after eight to 12 weeks, and then adjust the levels you supplement accordingly.

The ultimate aim of methylation is to liberate methyl groups and thereby give your brain the flexibility to adapt to changing circumstances. 'Methyl' nutrients such as TMG (tri-methyl-glycine), which provides three methyl groups, are classic examples of the nutrients that can improve methylation, but there are others. The vital phospholipid, phosphatidyl choline, which is very rich in eggs, also provides three methyl groups, and this may be another reason why this nutrient is coming up trumps for mental health. Another way to get a methyl group is to supplement methyl-B_{12} or methylfolate. These are a little more expensive as supplements but worth the difference. The better-quality homocysteine support supplements use one of these. You may also find a nutrient called glutathione or n-acetyl cysteine is included in some supplements. These also assist lowering the homocysteine level and improving methylation.

Nourishing H factor foods

The best place to start is to eat more of the foods rich in the nutrients I have discussed in this chapter. These foods are shown in the chart below.

Sources of foods containing the H factor nutrients

Methylation-friendly nutrients	Found in
B_2	eggs, almonds, whole grains, soya beans, spinach, mushrooms, milk, poultry, organ meats
B_6	whole grains, bananas
B_{12}	meat, fish, dairy products, eggs
Folic acid	green leafy vegetables
Zinc	oysters, nuts, seeds, fish
Magnesium	seeds and green leafy vegetables
TMG	whole grains, spinach, beetroot and other root vegetables

---

The methyl-friendly lifestyle

Improved methylation is not just about diet and supplements. There are many lifestyle factors that affect it, including smoking, drinking coffee and stress. All these factors raise homocysteine, whereas alcohol in strict moderation can lower it (although large amounts are bad news), and exercise tends to improve levels.[188] Following my mood-boosting low-GL diet is consistent with lowering homocysteine levels and improving methylation.

SUMMARY

Here are some guidelines that apply to us all:

- If you often feel tired and low, check your homocysteine level.
- If it's high (above 7), supplement specific amounts of B_2, B_6, B_{12}, folic acid, zinc and TMG.
- In any event, take a multivitamin every day that provides at least 200mcg folate, 10mcg B_{12}, 25mg B_6, 10mg B_2, 200mg of magnesium and 5mg zinc.
- Eat plenty of greens, beans, nuts and seeds for folate, and fish, meat, eggs or dairy products for their B_{12} content.
- Don't smoke.
- Minimise your intake of alcohol, coffee and caffeinated drinks.
- Minimise your stress.
- Keep fit.
- See Part 3 for your complete Mood-boosting Action Plan.

Chapter 14

VITAMIN D AND EXERCISE – A WINNING COMBINATION

From an evolutionary point of view we are all designed to be naked, living outdoors as hunter-gatherers and a lot further south than the UK. As a consequence, most of us in the northern hemisphere lack sufficient sunlight and exercise, especially in the winter.

One reason for feeling blue in the winter, according to research from the Baker Heart Research Institute in Melbourne, is that serotonin levels in the brain are lowest in the winter, and the amount of serotonin our brains produce is directly related to how much daylight we are exposed to.[189] So, with shorter days and less light, people with seasonal affective disorder, known as SAD, can really suffer. Some people, especially women, are prone to low levels of serotonin anyway, and a relative lack of light can tip them over the edge into depression. But there's another reason, and that is a lack of vitamin D. This vital mood-boosting vitamin is made in the skin in the presence of sunlight, and many of us, especially in the winter, don't make enough.

For these people, the symptoms of SAD usually recur regularly each winter and may include sleep problems, lethargy, overeating, social withdrawal, anxiety, loss of libido and mood changes. Most sufferers show signs of a weakened immune system during the winter, and are more vulnerable to infections and other illnesses. Some of these symptoms are associated with vitamin D deficiency and others with 'metabolic syndrome' (discussed in Chapter 7 in relation to keeping your blood sugar level even). Studies in Finland have shown that the worse the lighting at home the higher the incidence of symptoms of both metabolic syndrome and low mood.[190]

CASE STUDY: DARYL

> Daryl found that, particularly during the winter, he felt
> very low, irritable and angry, and was suffering from what
> he described as 'brain fog'. During the winter he would
> wake up feeling depressed, with a headache, and felt very
> lethargic. As a result, he would often have to take naps
> during the day. In the past he had taken various
> antidepressants; however, he didn't experience any relief
> from his symptoms.
>
> Daryl visited the Brain Bio Centre where tests revealed
> that he was low in vitamin D and essential fats. He was
> given a supplement programme to correct these
> deficiencies and he also began taking tryptophan. He
> quickly noticed what he described as a 'massive
> improvement' in his symptoms. He was no longer waking
> with headaches for the first time in six years, instead
> feeling refreshed with a clear mind. He also started to
> spend more time outdoors and felt his general well-being
> had greatly improved.

How to boost your serotonin levels

One way to counteract all this is to increase your exposure to light by spending more time outdoors, as Daryl did, or increasing your exposure to 'full spectrum' light. (Bear in mind that while sunlight exposure is very good for your mood, burning your skin is never good, so wear a good sunscreen if your skin will have longer periods of exposure to the sun. Also, try to keep out of intensive sunlight during the middle of the day.) Many studies have shown the effectiveness of bright light treatment with full-spectrum lights and what's called 'dawn simulation' for those with SAD. It has even been found that increasing bright light exposure for non-seasonal depression is as effective as antidepressants,[191] and even among those who do not suffer with seasonal mood swings as such.[192] The effect could be due to the direct effect of light on raising serotonin,[193] because light affects the pineal gland, which also produces serotonin's close relative, melatonin. A tryptophan-derived brain chemical, melatonin helps to balance the brain in the absence of light. Supplementing it has also proved helpful for those with SAD. Since melatonin is made from serotonin, and serotonin is made from 5-HTP (see illustration How the Brain Makes Melatonin on page 127), it is likely that, if you are prone to SAD, supplementing 5-HTP may help (see page 110).

Let there be light

How do you get more winter light without emigrating? Investing in a winter holiday in the sun is certainly one way; a less expensive alternative is investing in 'full-spectrum' lighting. These are light bulbs that have the same quality of light as the sun, determined by the spread of different wavelengths. That's why sunlight, and full-spectrum lighting, appears much whiter than a normal artificial light, which is yellower. Compared to ordinary bulbs, full-spectrum bulbs, although more expensive to start with, last ten times longer and use a quarter of the electricity, so they are also environmentally friendly.

During the winter, as it gets darker earlier in the evening, it helps to increase the intensity of light with a full spectrum light box. This boosts the light in any room you are in. If you have to wake up before it is light you can also use a 'dawn simulation' alarm. This is a bedside light that you set, much like an alarm clock, which simulates dawn light, with ever-increasing intensity until you wake up. In Resources I've listed the light products I prefer and the suppliers. In any event, it is best to maximise the available light by making sure that you are up at dawn during the autumn, winter and early spring. This may mean going to bed earlier if you are used to staying up late. (If you have difficulty getting to sleep, see Chapter 12.)

Alternatively, on the following page you'll find a simple exercise that takes one minute and involves a 60-watt light bulb, giving you an immediate serotonin boost.

EXERCISE: INCREASING YOUR EXPOSURE TO LIGHT

1 Sit down in a quiet place, on the floor or on a chair. It is best to choose a place that you can completely darken. If not, you will need a blindfold.

2 Place an anglepoise lamp with a 60-watt opaque (not clear) bulb, preferably with no writing on it, three feet away and directly in line with your line of vision.

3 Make sure you can turn the light on and off without moving your head position.

4 Turn the light on and look directly at the bulb for one minute, no longer. (You'll need a timer or watch for this.)

5 After one minute, turn the light off, close your eyes (put on your blindfold if the room is not completely dark) and focus on the after-image, the phosphene, without moving your head, until it completely vanishes. This usually takes three to four minutes.

6 This exercise is best done at dusk, effectively extending the daylight hours.

The vitamin D factor

Light has a direct effect on boosting the brain's feel-good neuro-transmitters, and it is also the most important way our body receives vitamin D. Although we take in some vitamin D from eating oily fish, and a little from eggs and milk, most of the vitamin D we receive comes from the conversion of cholesterol in the skin by sunlight. Most people in the northern hemisphere are deficient in vitamin D because of the lack of sun, particularly during the winter. The lower your vitamin D level the more likely you are to feel depressed and unmotivated. What is more, the darker your skin and the further you live from the equator the greater your risk will be of vitamin D deficiency.

One way of thinking of vitamin D is as a high-energy molecule. As I explained in Chapter 10 on essential fats, the sun's energy is absorbed into plankton in the seas, and from there into the little fish that feed on it. These in turn feed the carnivorous fish, such as mackerel and salmon. These 'oily' fish are the richest sources of vitamin D, along with fish liver oil such as cod liver oil. After the Second World War, when rickets caused by vitamin D deficiency was a major health issue, all children in Britain were given cod liver oil, providing not only vitamin D but also essential omega-3 fats and vitamin A. After supplementation was ceased, and combined with the decline in eating oily fish, vitamin D levels of people in the UK decreased and have done so ever since, with most people eating fewer than one serving of oily fish a week. The average woman in Britain achieves only 2.7mcg, while the average man achieves 3.1mcg, compared to the hopelessly low RDA of 5mcg. Many experts believe that we need as much as 30mcg a day in total.

Given that sunlight makes vitamin D, and a lack of sunlight is linked to feeling low, it is hardly surprising to find that low vitamin D levels in the winter is linked to low mood, but that doesn't prove that vitamin D deficiency is what 'causes' low mood. It might just be coincidental.

What the studies tell us

There is a growing body of research that not only links low vitamin D levels in the blood to a higher incidence of depression[194] but it also links them to premenstrual syndrome and seasonal affective disorder. The research shows that supplementing vitamin D and achieving optimal blood-vitamin D levels as a result also improves mood.

For example, researchers at the University of Tromso in Norway recruited 441 volunteers who were then given a test for depression and also a test for blood levels of vitamin D.[195] The lower the blood levels the higher was their depression rating. The volunteers were then given either 50mcg (2,000iu) of vitamin D or 100mcg (4,000iu) or placebo. After one year, those given vitamin D, but not those given the placebos, had lowered their depression ratings.

However, you don't have to wait for a year to get a lift in mood. A study in Australia involving 44 people found that those given vitamin D supplements (either 10mcg/400iu or 20mcg/800iu) had an improvement in mood in only five days compared to those not given vitamin D![196]

A small study in the US found a similar result. This involved nine women with low vitamin D levels (below 40ng/ml).[197] They were then given vitamin D, which resulted in a substantial decrease in their depression rating (by ten points) and an increase in their vitamin D levels by an average of 27ng/ml.

There's no doubt that more research is needed to firm up the evidence of vitamin D's mood-boosting effects but, to date, there is consistent evidence that those who are low in vitamin D benefit from supplementing more.

CASE STUDY: GABRIELLE

> Gabrielle came to the Brain Bio Centre in June 2009 suffering with extreme lethargy and mood swings. She would have to lie down for a few hours every day, and she found she had no energy to complete even the smallest of tasks.
>
> Tests showed a huge deficiency in vitamin D with low to borderline omega-3 and -6. Gabrielle then started a supplement programme to correct the deficiencies and almost immediately began to feel an improvement in her symptoms. Her energy levels increased substantially and she no longer had to rest every day. She is delighted with how she is now feeling and said:
>
> *'I've been trying to feel like this for 25 years, I'm over the moon!'*

How are your vitamin D levels?

The question you need to ask is, are you low in vitamin D and, if so, what's the best level to take in and how do you achieve this?

Vitamin D is easily tested by measuring the level of serum 25-hydroxyvitamin D (abbreviated to 25(OH)D). There's some debate about the exact level but, ideally, you are aiming for 125–200nmol/l (equivalent to 50–80ng/ml, which are the units of measurement used in the US). This is consistent with the levels found in people who live in sunny climates, and is consistent with the levels that correlate to the lowest risk of both depression and cancer (cancer incidence increases as you move away from the equator and is strongly linked to a lack of vitamin D). Below this level your body isn't storing vitamin D, which means that you are using it up as fast as you are taking it in. Since vitamin D is potentially toxic in very high levels, you don't want to have more.

Your vitamin D status is easily tested by your doctor or nutritional therapist.

What is your ideal level of vitamin D?

The next question is how much vitamin D do you need to take in to achieve your ideal level? This is harder to answer because, ideally, if you live in a sunny climate you'd make everything you need in your skin through sun exposure. It's the UVB rays that make vitamin D, which are also the rays that burn the skin. But obviously you need to avoid burning your skin. There's no advantage in that and you don't make more vitamin D as a result. Also, you can never 'overdose' on sun-produced vitamin D. The body simply makes what it needs.

If you live above or below 40 degrees north or south, however – which means all of Europe bar the tip of Spain and Italy – you won't get enough from sunlight all year round and will benefit from supplementation except during the summer months.

You need to supplement an absolute minimum of 12.5mcg (500iu) to guarantee a blood level of about 100nmol/l and probably more like 15mcg (600iu) to guarantee an ideal blood level above 125nmol/l.[198] That's what I take on a daily basis in my multivitamin supplement. That assumes you are getting a certain amount from your diet, plus sun exposure. We probably need more like 30–50mcg a day from all sources.

If you eat oily fish three times a week (a serving of salmon or mackerel provides around 9mcg/350iu); eat six free-range eggs a week (two eggs provide 1mcg/40iu); expose your skin to the sun every day (you'll make around 10mg/400iu if you have 20 minutes' exposure between 10 a.m. and 2 p.m. in the summer); and supplement at least 15mcg/600iu daily to give you around 30mcg/1,200iu a day. During the winter months (November to April in the UK) it's probably worth supplementing an additional 25mcg/1,000iu and possibly more, especially if you are older or prone to seasonal low moods.

How exercise helps too

If lack of sunlight and, consequently, a lack of vitamin D are two ways modern humankind has gone against our natural evolutionary design, exercise is another. When we were hunter-gatherers, exercise wasn't an option.

Exercise plays a key part in beating the blues. In fact, it turns out to be as effective as taking antidepressants. A number of studies in which people exercised for 30–60 minutes three to five times a week found a drop of around 5 points in their Ham-D score – more than double what you'd expect from antidepressants alone.[199] In an Australian study published in 2005 and involving 60 adults over the age of 60, half the volunteers took up high-intensity exercise three days a week, while the other half took low-intensity exercise. Of those taking high-intensity exercise, 61 per cent halved their Ham-D score, whereas only 29 per cent of those taking low-intensity exercise halved their score.[200] You've got to keep exercising to stay happy, however. An eight-year follow-up study of people prone to depression found that their depression returned if they stopped exercising.[201]

If you exercise outdoors, thereby combining exercising with sunlight exposure, that's all the better. In one study published in 2004, a third of depressed volunteers who exercised in full-spectrum lighting experienced a major improvement in their depression (a 50 per cent or more decrease in their Ham-D score).[202] Only 5 per cent of UVB rays, the ones that make vitamin D, get through glass so, when you can, exercise outdoors, not behind glass.

Exercise and sleep

Another advantage of exercise is that it helps you to sleep, which, as we saw in Chapter 12, is a big mood improver. A study of adolescent athletes found that they fell asleep faster, woke less frequently, were less tired, had increased concentration and reported significantly lower anxiety and fewer depressive symptoms.[203] Another study on older people found the same thing.[204] This may be because exercise helps to 'burn off' excess adrenalin and generally helps to stabilise blood sugar levels.

Getting motivated

Of course, one of the issues about exercising is that if you are feeling down and de-motivated it's not easy to get started, but the benefits are worth it. Also, once you begin my mood-boosting diet, and are taking the right supplements, you will experience a big improvement in energy levels, and exercise is a great way to expend it. Exercising also helps to balance blood sugar and therefore aids weight loss and that, in turn, improves your mood and motivation.

When you begin, aim for 20 minutes of exercise five days a week although, in truth, 30 minutes a day would be better. If you are significantly overweight this could be brisk walking. Find some exercise you like doing and other people to do it with; it's great to have an exercise buddy.

One of my favourite forms of exercise is Psychocalisthenics. This is a series of exercises that keeps you fit, strong and supple. It is also designed to generate vital energy – the life force or will to live, which fuels what you experience as energy, drive or enthusiasm. It definitely gives you a mood and energy lift and only takes 15–20 minutes a day to do. You can follow Psychocalisthenics from a DVD, but it's best to learn it in a half-day training session (see Resources).

SUMMARY

Here's what to do for a natural mood boost:

- Expose your skin to sunlight for 30 minutes a day with at least your face and arms exposed. But don't burn your skin.
- If you are prone to feeling low in the winter, invest in some full-spectrum lighting, and extend the length of your light exposure.
- Take a daily multivitamin that provides 15mcg (600iu) of vitamin D.
- Eat oily fish (fresh, canned or smoked salmon, mackerel, herring, kippers, sardines), which are rich in vitamin D, at least three times a week.

CONTINUED...

- During the winter take an additional vitamin D supplement providing 25mcg (1,000iu), especially if you are prone to low moods at that time of the year.
- Build exercise into your daily routine, for at least 20 minutes a day, preferably outdoors.
- See Part 3 for your complete Mood-boosting Action Plan.

Chapter 15

ST JOHN'S WORT: THE HAPPINESS HERB

A highly effective natural mood-boosting remedy is the herb St John's wort (*Hypericum perforatum*). It is one of the most thoroughly researched of all natural remedies.

St John's wort works just as well as tricyclic and SSRI antidepressants, but has fewer side effects. The older tricyclic antidepressants are still widely prescribed but often produce undesirable side effects; for example, in a study published in the *British Medical Journal*, 324 patients were randomly assigned to treatment with either St John's wort or the tricyclic antidepressant imipramine. Both were equally effective in treating patients with mild to moderate depression; however, St John's wort was better tolerated than imipramine and fewer patients withdrew as a result of adverse effects.[205]

An analysis of 29 such 'randomised' clinical trials on St John's wort versus placebos, involving 5,489 people in total, proves that the herb is highly effective with minimal side effects.[206] 'Both in placebo-controlled trials and in comparisons with standard antidepressants, trials from German-speaking countries reported findings more favourable to hypericum. Patients given hypericum extracts dropped out of trials due to adverse effects less frequently than those given older antidepressants', concludes this Cochrane systematic review. In one German study using 300mg of St John's wort, 66 per cent of patients with mild to moderate depression improved, with less depression and complaints of disturbed sleep, headache and fatigue, compared to just 26 per cent of those receiving a placebo.[207] It is not, however, as effective for severe depression. The same is true for SSRI antidepressants. German doctors frequently recommend St John's wort. UK doctors rarely do.

Are there any side effects?

One of the consistent findings in this research, and in my clinical experience, is that St John's wort has minimal side effects. It is much gentler than antidepressant drugs. That said, there are some side effects reported. About 2 per cent of people report side effects including gastrointestinal symptoms, allergic reactions, anxiety and dizziness. These have often been exaggerated in the media, possibly because more and more people are opting to take St John's wort instead of antidepressant drugs, and the drugs companies are fighting back with scare stories in the popular press.

Concerns about St John's wort causing photosensitivity (increased skin sensitivity to strong sunlight) should not be alarming, having only occurred at very high doses rather than the recommended 600–900mg a day.[208]

St John's wort does 'up regulate' certain liver enzymes. This means that the liver works a bit harder. The same happens with almost all drugs and substances foreign to the body, as the liver tries to detoxify them. It is therefore not advisable to combine St John's wort with SSRI antidepressants, anti-retroviral drugs or cancer drugs.[209]

Because of these kinds of concerns, St John's wort has been tested for long-term safety. In one study involving 440 people treated with St John's wort for a year, no significant side effects occurred, although there were a few reports of gastrointestinal side effects and the occasional skin complaint. The Ham-D score, however, dropped from an average of 20, indicating moderate depression, to an average of 2, indicating complete remission.[210] This and other research suggests that St John's wort is a much better and safer bet to continue long term to prevent a relapse of low mood than conventional antidepressants.[211]

The prominent psychiatrist Dr Hyla Cass is one of the world's leading experts on St John's wort. In her excellent book *St John's Wort: Nature's Blues Buster,* she gives ten reasons why she prefers St John's wort to antidepressant drugs:

1 Its side effects are not nearly as severe or frequent.

2 Mixing St John's wort with alcohol doesn't lead to adverse reactions, as with the other antidepressants.

3 It is not addictive.

4 It does not produce withdrawal symptoms when you stop.

5 It does not produce habituation, or the need for increased dosages to maintain its effects.

6 It can be easily stopped and restarted without requiring a long build-up period.

7 It enhances sleep and dreaming.

8 It does not inhibit sex drive as SSRIs do in some people – and can actually enhance it in some people.

9 It does not make you sleepy in the daytime. In fact, it has shown in experiments to enhance alertness and driving reaction time.

10 According to one report, the annual rate of death by overdose on antidepressant drugs is 30.1 per 1 million prescriptions. No one has ever died from an overdose of St John's wort. In fact, we don't think anyone has even tried to OD with it.

Do we know how it works?

Exactly how St John's wort works is still a bit of a mystery. Recent research indicates that hypericin, thought to be one of the major active ingredients in this herb, may act by inhibiting the reuptake of serotonin and dopamine. This may explain some of its benefits, but not all. In another study where the purported active ingredient hypericin was removed, St John's wort still raised levels of the brain chemicals. So we have to conclude that, so far, we still don't know enough about the activities and synergistic abilities of the many compounds found in St John's wort and exactly why it works.

How much should you take?

A 300mg dose of St John's wort (containing 0.3 per cent hypericin) two or three times a day helps most people with mild depression, while twice this amount (meaning 600mg three times a day) may help those who suffer severely. For the latter, buy a 450mg standardised St John's wort capsule. Take one on the first day, add a second dose at noon on the second day, then take a third dose on the next day, in the afternoon. If you have no adverse effects, you can take all three, 1,350mg, in the morning. But don't expect instant results. It often takes a couple of weeks to work. If you are currently on antidepressants I don't recommend also taking St John's wort, as not enough is known about their effects in combination.

SUMMARY

- Start taking a 300mg or 450mg dose of a standardised extract of St John's wort (containing 0.3 per cent hypericin) once a day and then increase to twice a day for a few days, then three times a day. Stop at the dose that makes you feel better. If you get any adverse effects, don't increase the dose.
- See Part 3 for your complete Mood-boosting Action Plan.

Chapter 16

ACCEPT AND MOVE THROUGH YOUR MOODS

The experience of life means that we inevitably accumulate emotional tension and unresolved memories from the past. The more disturbing of these become deep-rooted negative emotional patterns that unconsciously determine how we react to the stresses of life. When our life's circumstances change, it is completely natural, and healthy, to go through periods of low moods and depression, although it is important not to let these periods of low moods grow so that they dominate our life. This chapter is about how we can learn from the low times to enable us to make positive life changes.

The word 'emotion' comes from the Latin *emovere*: *e* for 'ex' or 'out' and *movere* for 'move', so emotion is a natural energy, a dynamic experience that needs to move through and out of the body. As children, however, we are often taught not to express our emotions; for example, we might have heard 'Don't be a cry-baby'. Or, when we are angry, we are taught it's not appropriate to express it: 'Calm down!' At some level most of us are taught that emotions are not OK; it is much easier in our society to say, for example, 'I have a stomach ache' than 'I am feeling depressed'.

As healthy adults, our task is to learn from the experiences of life and to let go of the emotional patterns from the past that mess up our lives and no longer serve us. As Fritz Perls, the founder of Gestalt Therapy often said, 'The only way out is through.' It's not easy, and the vast majority of people deny the symptoms or anaesthetise themselves through work, TV, food, alcohol or some kind of drug, including prescribed medication.

Our body expresses feelings we have repressed

These emotions literally store in our body's memory. That's why, when you recall an emotionally charged incident, it literally triggers that emotion again. They can manifest as physical tension, causing all kinds of health problems, including headaches, ulcers, IBS and more serious illnesses from cancer to cardiovascular disease. Extreme emotions affect your heart function, depress the immune system and inhibit digestion. In a state of depression the body's systems go haywire. Many people either lose lots of weight or they gain it. The body's repair mechanisms shut down; digestion gets worse; and if you also use toxic substances such as alcohol or sugar, or you are binge eating to numb whatever you are feeling, the body becomes overloaded with toxins. Sweating more and peeing frequently can be signs of this. Depression also depresses your immunity so that you become more prone to infections. This may be one explanation as to why many people who are unable to come to terms with the death of their partner often die shortly after.[212] Such emotions need to be fully expressed, for both our physical and psychological health, so that we can then learn from our experiences and move forward.

Anger, fear and sadness

We all experience many different emotions, but the most common ones are shades of anger, fear or sadness. Sadness is usually associated with regrets, losses and the loss of opportunities in the past. Anger is associated with not having our needs met, not being listened to, or not being understood. We also have sexual needs and the need for physical and emotional satisfaction and intimacy. Rage, violent reactions and extreme anger usually originate from a sense, whether real or just perceived, that our survival is literally under threat. Fear often comes from not being able to adapt to the circumstances we are in and is associated with the fear of our loss of our sense of self; for example, the fear of going mad or dying.

How do you relate to feelings?

What is it to have a healthy emotional response to life's inevitable circumstances? Aristotle said, 'Anyone can become angry – that is easy. But to be angry with the right person at the right time, for the right purpose, and in the right way – this is not easy.' How do you deal with a circumstance where someone accuses you of something you didn't do? Or when your relationship breaks down and ends, or when a loved one dies? How about when you lose your job or run out of money? Before exploring these questions it's good to have a brief emotional check-up to see how you relate to the world of feelings.

Questionnaire: check your emotional health

	Yes	No
1 Do you feel your emotions take over your life at times, or do you often feel disconnected from your emotions?	☐	☐
2 Are you often angry, upset, irritable, grumpy or feel aggressive?	☐	☐
3 How do you relate to anger?		
a Do you explode, shout and scream?	☐	☐
b Do you take it out on yourself by crying or putting yourself down, or do you deny it or never feel it?	☐	☐
c Do you rarely feel angry and express it appropriately when you do?	☐	☐
4 Are you often sad, suffering from mood swings or depression?	☐	☐
5 How do you relate to sadness?		
a Do you often cry and are you capable of crying for hours?	☐	☐
b Do you rarely let yourself feel it or deny it, perhaps saying that life is too short?	☐	☐
c When you feel sad, do you express it appropriately?	☐	☐

	Yes	No
6 Are you often fearful or anxious?	☐	☐

7 How do you relate to fear, such as a fear of change, abandonment/loss, fear of success or failure or poverty, ill health and death?

	Yes	No
a Are you often fearful about situations that have not happened?	☐	☐
b Do you find it difficult to let go of fears about things that have happened in the past?	☐	☐
c Are most of your fears justified and do you take appropriate action to move on?	☐	☐
8 Do you find it difficult to convey your feelings to others?	☐	☐
9 Do you find it difficult to express sadness, anger or fear?	☐	☐
10 Do you feel a lack of enough love in your life?	☐	☐
11 Do you find it difficult to spend time alone and try to avoid it?	☐	☐
12 Do you rarely reward or acknowledge yourself for your achievements?	☐	☐
13 Do you rarely feel completely content or happy?	☐	☐

14 How would you assess your relationship with your:

	Very good	Good	OK	Not good	Bad
Spouse/lover/partner (if you have one)	☐	☐	☐	☐	☐
Mother (if still alive)	☐	☐	☐	☐	☐
Father (if still alive)	☐	☐	☐	☐	☐
Brothers and sisters	☐	☐	☐	☐	☐
Friends	☐	☐	☐	☐	☐
Colleagues at work	☐	☐	☐	☐	☐
Self	☐	☐	☐	☐	☐

Score 1 point for each 'yes' answer; 2 points if you answered (a) in questions 3, 5 and 7, and 1 point if you answered (b); 2 points for any relationships you related as 'bad', and 1 point for any relationship you rated as 'not good'.

Total score:

Score

0–4
You have a high emotional IQ, reacting to situations appropriately, and effectively managing and enjoying your relationships.

5–7
You have signs of emotional issues that need some work. The recommendations in this chapter are likely to help.

8–12
You are in need of an emotional detox and are very likely to benefit a lot from some appropriate counselling. This chapter explains what works.

13 or more
Negative emotional patterns are having a major impact on the quality of your life and are likely to affect your health unless you deal with them now.

Depression is an opportunity

It may not seem like it, but feeling depressed is an opportunity. If you read autobiographies of great and interesting people, they all go through periods of depression. The trick is not to get stuck by avoiding the underlying issues that bring on the feelings of being low and thinking that there is no point or meaning to life. This, after all, is the main symptom of deep depression: the feeling that there is no point, and no meaning and that nothing interests you. Other common attributes are feeling anxious, fearful, angry and irritable.

This can actually be a useful place to be if you know how to work it. If this is how you feel right now, two excellent books to read are Thomas

Moore's *Dark Nights of the Soul* and *Care of the Soul*. It is important to recognise these times and to accept them for what they are trying to tell us, however painful they may be, because it is through these dark passages that we come into deeper levels of understanding about who we are and our purpose in life. So, the essential point is not to resist them, but to honour them as part of the cycle of life. There is no shortcut. Without purpose and a real sense of who we are, life is depressing.

What are you missing?

For many, depression is really mourning something or someone that has been lost. This could be a missed opportunity, a lost relationship, the death of a friend, a pet, the death of a dream or the loss of a way of life you've become accustomed to. Many people struggle with retirement precisely because they lose a way of life that has become a habit, and lose their position or place in a team. For others a change in circumstances means a loss of the sense of being in control, which is, at one level, an illusion because nothing stays the same.

If you are depressed, ask yourself what have been the big changes in your life since you started to feel low? When you know what you are missing – for example, a friend, a job or a dream – ask yourself what quality is now missing from your life? What is it about whatever you are missing that you miss the most? It could be a routine, companionship or a nurturing environment.

Feeling trapped

Another common theme in depression is feeling trapped by one's circumstances and somehow blaming those circumstances for not allowing you to be who you really are. In this sense you may be betraying yourself by staying in a job or a relationship, or not taking up an opportunity that is true to who you really are.

We are creatures of habit and we do become attached to a particular sense of identity. When that identity gets shattered in some way, we are left with a loss of the sense of self. With that comes a loss of purpose or meaning.

The meanings in our lives

At different times in our life we create meaning in different ways. One way to explore this is to write down as many possible meanings or identities you could have or have had; for example, I am 'the house I live in'; I am 'the clothes I have'; I am 'the money I've made'. Perhaps, when you were younger your goal was to meet the right man or woman, get married, have kids, and live in a lovely house. But you've done that, and the kids have left home and you are left feeling down and wondering what it's all about. Or perhaps you set your sights on a particular degree or career and didn't make the grades. Think of all the things that define you, or that you identify with, from your status – perhaps as a mother, father, wife or husband – to your handbag or iPhone. Write down as many as you can think of.

So often we have a dream, perhaps to set up house or attain a particular level at work, or to do something like writing a book or making money, or running a business and, in the process, our identity or sense of meaning becomes tied up in this. We might be attached to our position or stature but if we suffer a demotion, humiliation or defeat it is very painful to us. Of course, these things are not really *who* you are, but if your circumstances change you can end up unsettled and depressed, mourning something that was there before but isn't there anymore.

How can you move on?

This first step, that of recognising and acknowledging what it is you are missing, isn't easy, and good counsellors and good friends can help you see what the fundamental issues are when you feel lost. As King Lear says in Shakespeare's play, 'Who is it who can see me and tell me who I am?' It's incredibly helpful to find someone whom you trust who sees you for who you are. In Resources you will find details on how to find a psychotherapist or counsellor, but the most important thing is to have someone to talk to who really understands who you are beyond the ups and downs of life.

One way to work through your thoughts on your own is to try free-association journaling. To do this, set aside exactly 20 minutes a day, ideally in the morning, when you can just write down whatever comes into your mind non-stop for 20 minutes. You'll often be surprised by what comes out, which will help you to realise the real issues fuelling your low moods.

Mind over moods

When you are feeling low, it's very hard to have a perspective on things. In fact, the tendency is to view everything as much worse than it is. We start to buy into all sorts of negative thoughts. Here are some of the common ones:

The automatic thoughts of people who are depressed:

1 I feel like I'm up against the world.

2 I'm no good.

3 Why can't I ever succeed?

4 No one understands me.

5 I've let people down.

6 I don't think I can go on.

7 I wish I were a better person.

8 I'm so weak.

9 My life's not going the way I want it to.

10 I'm so disappointed in myself.

11 Nothing feels good anymore.

12 I can't stand this anymore.

13 I can't get started.

14 What's wrong with me?

15 I wish I were somewhere else.

16 I can't get things together.

17 I hate myself.

18 I'm worthless.

19 I wish I could disappear.

20 What's the matter with me?

21 I'm a loser.

22 My life's a mess.

23 I'm a failure.

24 I'll never make it.

25 I feel so helpless.

26 Something has to change.

27 There must be something wrong with me.

28 My future is bleak.

29 It's just not worth it.

30 I can't finish anything.

('Automatic Thoughts Questionnaire' copyright 1980 by Philip C. Kendall and Steven D. Hollon. Reprinted by permission.)

How many of the above hold true for you? To add insult to injury we often get depressed about being depressed. The psychologist Roberto Assagioli, who developed an excellent psychotherapy approach called psychosynthesis, describes this as 'building a two storey building'. All emotional states change, but when you feel low you project that you'll feel this way for ever and imagine everything – your job, relationships and so on – coming to an end. In fact, it becomes impossible to see that these transitional phases often have great blessings, and offer openings into new opportunities at the end. But, when you feel low you probably imagine that the light at the end of the tunnel is a freight train rapidly approaching, as you clutch on to that which is familiar, but no longer serves you or is there for you.

Cognitive behavioural therapy, or CBT, addresses how negative thoughts perpetuate feelings and unhelpful behaviours. It focuses on specific ways to change the way you think which, in turn, changes how you feel. CBT is one of the most widely used psychotherapeutic techniques that help you move through low moods. If you would like to explore it for yourself read *Mind over Mood* by Dennis Greenberger and Christine Padesky. This is really a workbook that takes you through the process. Many psychotherapists and counsellors use CBT in their approach, which has proven highly effective, as has psychotherapy in general, in lessening depression.[213] People who have received CBT are almost half as likely to relapse into depression as those who have taken antidepressant medication only.[214] If you think you would benefit from CBT with a therapist, you can request this from your doctor, although you may have to wait for some time, as there are not enough therapists to meet the demand.

Developing mindfulness

One step on from this is an approach, now widely practised by psychotherapists in one form or another, called MBT – mindfulness behavioural therapy. This can be very effective in helping you to find your way back to your true sense of self by allowing you to witness your thoughts, feelings and physical sensations, thereby allowing them to transform. There's growing evidence, not only that this approach is highly effective[215] but also that developing mindfulness actually changes brainwave patterns towards alpha and theta waves, which are consistent with a more relaxed and creative way of being.[216]

Of course, this isn't easy to do to start with, but Rome wasn't built in a day, and simple exercises or a therapy session can be very helpful. The book *The Mindful Way Through Depression* by Mark Williams, John Teasdale, Zindel Segal and Jon Kabat-Zinn, which also contains a CD, takes you through such exercises in a well-explained way.

You can start by being mindful of your feelings. As the authors say:

Each emotion is a full-body reaction to a characteristic situation: fear is triggered when danger threatens: sadness and grief when something precious is lost; disgust when something unpleasant is confronted; anger when an important goal is blocked; happiness when our needs are met. Naturally they tell us what to do to survive and even thrive ... The problem is we try to think our way out of our moods by working out what's gone wrong. Unfortunately, these critical thinking skills might be exactly the wrong tools for the job.

A more mindful way is to 'honour' your feelings and allow yourself to feel them without judgemental thoughts. One way to do this, which is especially helpful if you find it hard to identify what you are feeling, is to put your awareness into the physical sensation:

1 Where in your body do you feel it?

2 What is that physical sensation actually like?

Breaking the cycle

Mindfulness, the authors define as 'the awareness that emerges through paying attention on purpose, in the present moment, and non-judgementally to things as they are'.

The trouble is that we get caught in this cycle of thoughts–feelings–physical sensations–behaviours. The purpose of mindfulness is to break this automatic cycle that reinforces a pattern which keeps you feeling depressed, anxious and exhausted. Thoughts are just thoughts. They aren't real as such – they are just interpretations. We automatically try to avoid uncomfortable feelings or physical sensations, but by acknowledging them, experiencing them, breathing into them – which means experiencing the feeling in your body and literally breathing deeply into it – and allowing them to exist, they do naturally change. Resisting negative feelings is what makes them persist.

If you like the sound of mindfulness, find a counsellor who practises MBT or read the book *The Mindful Way Through Depression*. Another excellent book, and approach, that helps to bring you into a state of mindfulness is Eckhart Tolle's *Power of Now*.

Freeing your thoughts

One way to improve your mood and bring you into a more mindful state is to go for a walk outside, perhaps in your local park. The simple act of focusing on what is going on in the world around you can help to bring you out of your incessant negative thought patterns. Exercise is also excellent because you have to focus on your physical movement and body, with little time to think. (That's apart from the endorphin effect that we explored in Chapter 14.) Listening to music is also good, and Mozart in particular comes highly recommended; his music has been shown to improve brainwave patterns. Learning something is also an effective way to come back into your self. People who are stuck in depression often find it very hard to learn, but the exercise of learning something new can be very helpful.

There are other ways of entering into a state of mindfulness, which is really the purpose of most meditative techniques. While meditation has many proven health benefits, the real purpose is to bring you back to your true self, able to witness changing moods and thoughts, rather than becoming lost in them. Many yoga classes also introduce you to basic meditation techniques and can be very uplifting. One meditation technique is called Holosync, which involves just sitting and listening to a meditative CD that very specifically changes your brainwave patterns into a mindful state (alpha and theta waves) and away from negative thought patterns. It is highly effective for some people (see Resources for details). In Chapter 12 I told you about the work of John Levine and his CD *Silence of Peace*. Listening to the CD helps to move your brainwave patterns into the alpha state, which is more consistent with mindfulness.

What do you enjoy doing?

If all the above seems too much, a quick way to break a pattern of depressive thoughts is simply to do something you enjoy. Often, when we feel particularly low we feel like we don't enjoy anything and just want to hide away. Do something, anything, you enjoy, whether it's big or small – even if it's something that's nutritionally not 'good' for you. It might be drinking a hot chocolate, or going to the movies, travelling, or having a massage or stroking your cat. These simple acts are acts of kindness to yourself. So too is giving yourself good nutrition. Buying healthy food and making yourself something simple, maybe a healthful soup, is a simple act of kindness for your body.

Finding your self

Ultimately, the way up from down is about finding yourself, and techniques such as mindfulness give you the internal space to do just that. The job of a counsellor or psychotherapist is to help you find your sense of self – who you really are – and help you discover your sense of purpose.

Reconnecting with your self and sense of purpose is the mission of Byron Katie. In her excellent book *Who Would You Be Without Your Story?* she takes you through a powerful process whereby you ask yourself four questions about any particular thought; for example, if you've split up with your partner and are mourning that loss you may have the thought, *I want my husband/wife back.* Katie asks us to examine that thought by asking four questions:

1 Is it true?

2 Do I absolutely know that it is true?

3 How do I react when I think that thought?

4 Who would I be without the thought?

Much like the mindfulness approach I spoke about earlier, Katie talks about how the nature of our minds is to have thoughts and to validate what we believe. That's what the mind does. Thoughts can be wonderful, or they can be terribly destructive. Our mind can find reasons why we are justified in feeling the way we do, and in blaming others, but this kind of reasoning doesn't generally make us happy and it fuels negative emotions and stress. If we believe something that isn't true for us, a feeling will let us know (and a healthy diet plus all the mood-boosting omega-3 in the world won't change that feeling). That is why it is so important to question our thoughts and beliefs. If we don't, life will challenge us. That is why every apparent tragedy and loss in life really is an opportunity to grow and learn.

Getting the past out of the present

Of course, the big problem with any concept of being fully present in the moment is that we have history. We get stuck in negative emotional and behavioural patterns. A good friend or therapist can act as a mirror, helping to make us aware of negative patterns of behaviour, which are like the traps we keep falling into. But how do you break free? Simply feeling something fully, and noticing negative patterns, gives you the distance to become free of them. You don't necessarily have to 'do' something.

When you react emotionally, these reactions are automatic and physical, literally flooding your brain and body with neurotransmitters associated with the stress response. They take over your rational mind, stop you being able to listen and lead to irrational reactions and behaviour. Your heart rate can jump from 70 beats a minute to over 100 in a single heartbeat, your muscles tense and your breathing changes.

Daniel Goleman, author of *Emotional Intelligence*, calls this 'emotional hijacking'.[217] These emotional-reaction patterns that trigger emotional hijacking are learned in early life and can be changed into more functional responses by coming to an understanding of how our past programmes us to respond automatically to current events.

How do you deal with anger and sadness?

As an example, cast your mind back to your early childhood. How did you see anger expressed in your childhood? Did you ever see your mother or father shouting, or did they give you the silent treatment? You were able to sense their anger underneath. What did you learn from this? If you had a raging, shouting parent, you've probably learned to shut down, as you had to do when you were a frightened and vulnerable child. Perhaps you said that you'd never be like that when you grew up, and swore that you would certainly never ever treat your children in that way. Yet, in a moment of weakness or frustration, you might have reacted in just the same way they did, and felt really guilty afterwards. It can take a lot of energy to be different from how we were brought up, because we have had years of 'emotional education', both positive and negative, from our parents as well as our schoolteachers.

A softer emotion than anger is sadness. Think back to how your parents dealt with sadness or grief; for example, if there was a death in the family, how did your parents react? Sadness is an appropriate reaction, but left unexpressed, it leads to depression.

Depression can arise from suppressed anger. 'Don't get sad, get mad' the saying goes. If you are depressed, is there something you are angry about but have been unable to express or do something about? Do you think either of your parents was depressed and, if so, how has this affected you? Are you either always trying to be positive about everything or do you have an underlying sense of hopelessness, or perhaps you flip-flop between the two?

Your relationships

Do you fear that any love relationships are doomed, a minefield that could explode at any time or are best avoided completely? What lessons did you learn about love and relationships when you were growing up? If you always fear being abandoned or not finding a loving relationship, that may very well stem from early memories of feeling abandoned or unwanted as a child.

The kind of relationship your parents had with each other will also have had a massive impact on how you deal with relationships. Here's an exercise that can help you see how we inherit these negative emotional patterns from our parents.

EXERCISE: IDENTIFYING YOUR NEGATIVE EMOTIONAL PATTERNS OF BEHAVIOUR

1 Write down at least five of your negative emotional patterns – ideally those that cause, or have caused you, the most emotional distress. Here are some examples:

- Fear of being abandoned (leads to being needy or clingy).
- Fear of being smothered in a relationship (leads to avoiding committed relationships).
- Feeling put down or criticised (leads to not taking risks).
- Feeling that you're never good enough (leads to having to achieve or prove yourself, or having to please).
- Feeling controlled (leads to having to control others).
- Feeling ashamed or guilty.
- Fear of being wrong (leads to having to be right).
- Fear of failure, or not making it in the world (leads to constant striving and over-achieving).

2 Now take a few moments to relax and take your mind back to a time in your childhood. Close your eyes and picture yourself as a child of around eight years old. You might even have a photo lying around that could help you access that picture. Standing next to yourself as a child, imagine your parents, or the people who brought you up, just as they were when you were growing up. Next to them, how do you feel? Are you given the sense that you are good enough, that you are OK as you are? Can you start to get the sense of how your whole mood, your attitude to others, indeed your overall perspective of the world might have been affected by these powerful figures? Remember, you depended on them for love and approval.

3 Now write down five or more negative patterns of your mother and your father. Look for the ones that had the most impact on you; for example: over-critical, uncaring, cold/distant, smothering, over-protective, angry, passive, hopeless.

4 Do any of the patterns you identified for yourself exist also in either of your parents? Or do you have the opposite pattern of behaviour? In many cases we compensate with the exact opposite; for example, your parent is aggressive, and you are passive, or they are critical and you are always nice.

Stopping the pattern from repeating

The real destructive power of the past can often come about because, despite our best intentions, we keep recreating history by subconsciously setting up situations that feel familiar. It's horrifying and strangely comforting at the same time. For example, if we had a critical parent we attract a critical partner or boss. Or if one of your parents was always blaming the other one for his or her problems, perhaps you have inherited the victim role. It's never your fault, and you always have someone else to blame. That's the power these negative patterns have in our lives. Psychologists call this 'transference' whereby we bring our internalised parents, along with their and our shared emotional baggage from the past, into our present lives.

Often, unconsciously, we hang on to a familiar, but potentially destructive type of relationship with our parents, or indeed a significant other. If you do get stuck in depression, a good question to ask yourself is: what primary relationship are you unwilling to let go of? Is it time to grow up, to stop blaming others and assume responsibility for yourself?

So, what do you do when you become aware of how learned negative emotional patterns are messing up your life and your health? In the same way that we need to learn about optimum nutrition and how to choose the right foods and drinks to be healthy, we also need to learn about how to discharge and let go of negative emotions and emotional patterns. As vital as this skill is, it unfortunately isn't taught in school and it isn't part of our culture to learn these things. The first step is to recognise and acknowledge how you feel in the moment.

Getting help

One of the most powerful and effective courses I have come across is a one-week residential course called the Hoffman Process. It thoroughly 'undoes' negative patterns of behaviour we inherit from childhood, resulting in a profound transformation in relating and relationships, and the sense of who we are. It crosses the fine line between psychology (healing the psyche) and spirituality – getting you back in touch with the higher self and the natural feeling of love that lies behind the feelings and thoughts we become trapped in. Participants report benefits such as much better relationships with family members and being able to communicate more effectively at home and at work. I often get letters from people who want to express their gratitude for the introduction to this excellent course, and the transformation they have received from doing it. (See Resources for details.) We run half-day workshops called Getting Your Past out of Your Present to introduce some of the techniques that form part of the Hoffman Process (see the events section at www.patrickholford.com).

Re-wiring your emotional brain

While the Hoffman Process is certainly a fast track to breaking deep-rooted destructive emotional patterns, the critical issue is how do we literally change the way we respond emotionally? One of the most insightful ways of understanding emotional patterns is via a process called Emotional Brain Training, or EBT.

EBT is rooted in the emerging understanding of exactly how the brain becomes 'wired' for certain emotional reactions. Much of this wiring is laid down very early in life. For example, if a baby is abandoned by its mother, its emotional brain (the limbic brain) reacts to the denial of this fundamental need by screaming and raging. If the mother returns and comforts the baby, its higher brain centre (the neocortex) learns that if it rages and hollers it receives love. The first track is laid down. If that pattern gets repeated again and again then any stimulus that triggers the emotional reaction associated with abandonment will result in the same pattern of reaction. It's literally part of the survival programming of the brain.

EBT focuses on how to change that wiring but it's important to understand that we have five basic levels of being or reacting. The example I just described is Brain State 5. Quoting from Laurel Mellin's excellent book *Wired for Joy* (see Resources):

'**In Brain State 5** you feel overwhelmed and confused, unable to think clearly, panicked, deeply depressed, even lost, and feel like you have always been this way and will always be this way – you are in a full-blown stress response.

In Brain State 4 you are definitely stressed, you aren't sure what to expect or your expectations are too harsh or too lenient and your negative feelings are rather intense.

In Brain State 3 you are a little stressed, still feel somewhat secure in your connection to yourself, but either have no feelings (numb) or a fair intensity of negative feelings.

In Brain State 2 you feel balanced and good, aware of both positive and negative feelings, and feel present in the moment.

In Brain State 1 you feel great and balanced with positive feelings, such as ripples of pleasure or the glow of wellbeing in your body. Or you feel calm and energised with a sense of purpose.'

The purpose of EBT is to help you identify which brain state you are in so that you can apply specific tools to help move you up the ladder towards Brain State 1, where you experience joy. Obviously, if you have clicked into a full-blown emotional reaction (Brain State 5) in which you feel utterly worthless and imagine you will always feel like this, meditation isn't going to help. By recognising that this is actually a pre-wired brain reaction the best you can do is not judge yourself (and others) too harshly, minimise the harm you create for yourself and others when in this state, and know that it will pass.

The wonder of EBT is that it gives you very specific tools for moving through these brain states and, most importantly, laying down new 'tracks' so that you gradually start to react to inevitable button-pushing events in a different way. There's a whole on-line community of people, and support tools, applying EBT methods (see www.ebt.org). We also run half-day workshops introducing the EBT approach (see events at www.patrickholford.com).

We all have a purpose

The common thread in low moods is losing one's sense of purpose, which is a key attribute of Brain State 1. By working through negative thoughts and feelings, and becoming more in touch with who you are, your purpose in life naturally emerges. In my book *The Ten Secrets of 100% Healthy People*, which explores the key qualities of super-healthy people, finding your purpose is the tenth secret. Here is one of the useful exercises that may help you become clearer on your purpose in life. You'll need a pen and some pieces of paper and a place to sit quietly and comfortably. (We also run workshops on purposeful living – see the events section on www.patrickholford.com.)

EXERCISE: FINDING YOUR PURPOSE

Exercise 1

1 Sit comfortably in a quiet place. Recollect how you felt at the age of ten. What gave you your sense of purpose then? What was your sense of purpose at ages 15, 20, 26 and 35? Write down whatever comes to mind without too much deliberation, making a list of different purposes you've been aware of at different times in your life.

2 Ask yourself, 'What gives me a sense of purpose now?' Write down as many of your current purposes as you can.

3 Now become still, focusing on your breath, and ask your innate wisdom, your higher intelligence, 'What is my true purpose?' Offer this question without 'thinking' the answer, and write down, without censorship, whatever comes to mind, starting with the words, 'My purpose in life is . . .'

Exercise 2

Another way to become clearer on your purpose is to answer these three questions:

1 What do you love to do or enjoy doing? What makes you feel good? What gives you a sense of satisfaction and fulfilment?

2 What are you good at? We all have certain gifts or talents. For some it's the ability to listen; for others it's having a clear mind. What are some of your gifts?

3 What is needed now in the world, in your community or your family? How can you use your gifts to help or to serve?

When you contemplate these three questions, and put the answers together, you will find powerful insights into your own purpose.

Discover your special gifts and enjoy giving

You are unique and you have your own unique gifts. The secret is to know what your gifts are and to give them. A deep sense of fulfilment can come from doing small things with love, and from expanding your circle of caring. Sometimes we feel we have gifts but we have no way to give them, or that they are not being received. Perhaps you are a great listener but your career gives you little opportunity to help people in this way. Then the question becomes: how can you give your gifts and fulfil your purpose in another context?

Those who have a sense of purpose and fulfilment usually have more connection with that part of themselves that is deeper than the thinking mind – and a larger circle of caring or expressing love.

All you need is love

Ultimately, there is nothing more important than love, especially in those times when you are going through a difficult transition. Sometimes we feel incapable of loving or that we are unlovable. It's easy to forget those friends who are there for us, and sometimes we can take advantage of their friendship by loading our troubles on them. But it is a great blessing if you have friends who love you for who you are, and have faith in you but who can also recognise your autonomy and that you have your own choices to make. Such friends will be there for you whatever happens. That is why it is important to build a relationship with someone you can trust, be it a therapist, a healthcare practitioner, a friend or your partner – or even your dog. We all need to feel loved and to express love. That, I believe, is what lies beyond our limited thoughts. It is the essential ground of being human.

The need to love and be loved is fundamental to all of us – more important than any vitamin. It is important to find a purpose that somehow expresses love or caring for others in whatever way that might be, and it is a critical piece of the Feel Good Factor.

PSYCHOLOGICAL HELP

Just as one might have an accountant or plumber to call on when issues arise, it is very helpful to have a psychotherapist or counsellor that you can touch base with when you hit a bad patch. As we have seen above, there are many different, and effective, psychotherapy approaches but, quite frankly, the most important thing is to find someone you click with and can trust; someone who can start to build an understanding of you, your life's influences and issues. In Resources I list organisations that have directories of local therapists, but it is also good to get recommendations. Your doctor or GP practice can also help. Psychotherapy is available on the NHS, although there is a waiting list.

Most psychotherapists will offer an initial meeting so that you can both feel happy that you can work with each other. This is a very important relationship and it's vital that you have a good rapport with your chosen therapist.

Living and learning through change

Life is a journey and one that always gives opportunities for learning and growing. Change is a vehicle for growth, and growth inevitably means pain, because most of us find change difficult. The only person who likes change is a baby in a wet nappy. No one can change you. In the end you are the only person who can change yourself. It is completely healthy to go through periods of depression or feeling low. Such times teach us how to let go of things and to learn from the rich experiences of life, however unpleasant they may sometimes be. The trick is not to get lost for too long along the way.

SUMMARY

Here are some things you can do for yourself:

- If you are feeling low, do something you like doing.
- Nourish yourself well. Eat healthy food and take your supplements every day.
- Go for walks and engage in physical activities.
- Talk to someone you trust who sees who you really are, beyond your ups and downs.
- Find a therapist you can work with, and touch base when you are going through difficult patches.
- Read a book that teaches you something about yourself (see Recommended Reading).
- Develop the art of mindfulness, meditation or EBT, of being rather than doing, be it via a book, a therapist or by attending a course or workshop.
- Explore what you need to live a life with purpose.
- See Part 3 for your complete Mood-boosting Action Plan.

Part Three

YOUR MOOD-BOOSTING ACTION PLAN

In this part I explain the nuts and bolts of your mood-lifting low-GL diet, including details of how to lose weight if you need to. You will also find full details of your supplement programme, depending on your particular needs, as highlighted by the results of the questionnaires you completed in Part 2. The part finishes with a blueprint for having a good day, including advice on how to start on a bright note and keep your mood lifted throughout.

Chapter 17

GOOD MOOD FOODS

By now you are well aware that a whole host of nutrients in food play a large part in making you feel good, and other foods can contribute to making you feel bad. But how do you put this all together so that you know what to buy and what to prepare for meals?

That's the purpose of this chapter. But before we get down to the practical issues, I'd like to show you the actual results of our 100% Health Survey on 55,570 people, looking closely at which food groups were associated with a good or bad 'mind and mood' score. Among those with a low mind and mood score, a little more than half (55 per cent) reported frequent or occasional anxiety, and almost half of the respondents reported depression, which may or may not have been clinically diagnosed.

What we then did was to look at the relationship between the consumption of different food groups in relation to the chances of having a very good or bad mind-and-mood rating. The results confirm other findings that some foods are positively good for helping to lift you out of depression and low moods, whereas others are best avoided because they can have a lowering effect on the mind. This is good news, because it means that by making simple changes to your diet you can look forward to improving your mood, not just now but always.

The bad and the good

The worst food group in our survey was sugary snacks, with high sugar-based snack consumption (three or more sugary snacks a day) almost doubling the likelihood of poor mind and mood health. This tallies with the link, shown in Chapter 7, between blood sugar problems, energy and mood. Next came high wheat consumption (five or more servings a day) – the more you eat the less is your chance of having a good mood rating. Compared to other food groups, the impact of negative foods was relatively greater than that of positive foods, suggesting that the foods you avoid that are bad for you will have more impact on your mood than increasing those foods that are good for you. Obviously, the ideal is to do both.

The most positive 'food' of all was water, followed by fresh fruit and oily fish – which makes sense in the context of omega-3s and vitamin D, both of which are rich in fish.

Food intake associated with poor mind and mood health

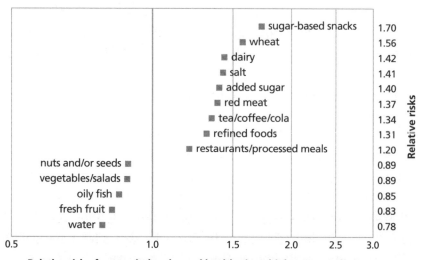

Relative risk of poor mind and mood health given high consumption

Any relative risk score below 1 means a reduced risk. A score above 1 means an increased risk. A score of 2 would mean double the risk. A high consumer of sugar-based snacks, at 1.7, is therefore getting close to doubling their risk of poor mental health.

The Feel Good Diet

The diet that follows contains all the foods necessary for general health, and it is also highly appropriate for those who suffer from low mood, because it contains those foods that are especially rich in the nutrients needed by the brain and avoids the mood-lowering 'danger' foods. It is based on the following principles:

Basic principles of the diet

- Carbohydrates should have a low-glycemic load (low-GL) to keep your blood sugar level even and minimise blood sugar dips.
- Wheat and milk – the two foods that most commonly cause allergic symptoms – are decreased and replaced with wheat- and dairy-free options.
- Sufficient protein is included to give you a good supply of amino acids.
- It is high in foods rich in B vitamins, such as beans, nuts and seeds, as well as green leafy vegetables, which are also rich in zinc and magnesium, to enhance methylation.
- It is high in essential omega-3 fats and vitamin D.

This means that you should include a serving of each of the following foods in your diet every day:

1 Fish, especially oily fish such as salmon, mackerel, herring, kippers, sardines and tuna (fresh); or free-range or organic eggs; or lean free-range chicken.

2 Nuts and seeds – especially chia seeds, flax seeds, pumpkin seeds, almonds and peanuts – and all beans (cannellini, red kidney, chickpeas, black-eyed beans, lentils, and so on).

3 Berries, cherries, plums, apples and pears.

4 Green vegetables (broccoli, kale, cabbage, watercress, rocket, asparagus, peas, artichoke).

But the single most important principle for keeping your mood and energy good is keeping your blood sugar level even by following a low-GL diet.

How to master your blood sugar by eating low GL

The reason I want you to focus on the carbohydrate content of foods is because the other two main food types – fat and protein – don't have any appreciable effect on your blood sugar. In fact, I recommend you eat some fat and protein *with* your carbohydrate, because this will further lessen the effect the carbohydrate has on your blood sugar, thereby lowering the glycemic load of the meal.

So, for balancing your blood sugar, there are only four rules:

Rule 1 Eat 40 GLs (explained below) a day to lose weight, and 60 to maintain it.

Rule 2 Eat carbohydrate with protein.

Rule 3 Graze don't gorge.

Rule 4 Cut back on stimulants.

The glycemic load (GL) is a precise measure of what effect a food has on your blood sugar balance (see box opposite). The examples of meals given in this chapter are based on 40 GLs a day (plus 5 GLs for drinks or a dessert): the amount needed to lose weight. If you don't need to lose weight, then you don't need to be so strict on the carbohydrate portions.

All animal produce, plus any type of seed, nut or bean is protein. Combining, for example, nuts with fruit, or egg with toast, fulfils the second rule of eating carbohydrate with protein and this helps to keep your blood sugar level for even longer.

The third rule means eating little and often. So, always eat breakfast, lunch and supper – and introduce a snack mid morning and mid afternoon. This way you'll provide your body with a constant and even supply of fuel, which means you'll experience fewer food cravings.

The fourth rule is especially important if you are in the habit of drinking coffee with a carbohydrate snack, such as a croissant. According to research at Canada's University of Guelph, this is a deadly duo as far as your blood sugar is concerned. Participants were given a carbohydrate snack, such as a croissant, a muffin or toast, together with either a decaf or caffeinated coffee. Those having the caffeine–carb combo had triple the increase in blood sugar levels, while insulin sensitivity was almost halved.[218]

I'd like to take you through a typical day, starting with breakfast, so that you get a good idea of how to apply these rules in your daily life. But first, it's worth understanding what glycemic load means and which kinds of foods are high or low GL.

UNDERSTANDING THE GLYCEMIC LOAD

The glycemic load combines the glycemic index with the concept of measuring carbohydrate intake to provide a scientifically superior way of controlling blood sugar. Put simply, the glycemic index (GI) of a food tells you whether the carbohydrates in the food are fast or slow releasing. It's a 'quality' measure. It doesn't tell you, however, how much of the food is carbohydrate. On the other hand, carbohydrate points, or grams of carbohydrate, tell you how much of the food is carbohydrate, but they don't tell you what that particular carbohydrate does to your blood sugar. This, therefore, is a 'quantity' measure. The glycemic load (GL) of a food is the quantity × the quality. It's the best way of judging if a particular food can make you gain weight.

Here are some examples of high- and low-GL carbohydrates, so that you can understand which types of foods to choose. Ideally, you want to eat 5 GLs for a snack and 7–10 GLs for the carbohydrate portion of a main meal. The low-GL foods are shown in **bold** and the high GL foods are shown in *italics*. (Note that protein and fat foods have no affect on your blood sugar, so are not shown in this list.)

Food	serving looks like	GLs
FRUIT		
Blueberries	**1 large punnet (600g)**	**5**
Apple	**1 small (100g)**	**5**
Grapefruit	**1 small**	**5**
Apricot	**4 apricots**	**5**

CONTINUED...

Food	serving looks like	GLs
Grapes	**10 grapes**	**5**
Pineapple	**1 thin slice**	**5**
Banana	*1 small banana*	*10*
Raisins	*20 raisins*	*10*
Dates	*2 dates*	*10*

STARCHY VEGETABLES

Pumpkin/squash	**1 large serving** (185g/6³/₄oz)	**7**
Carrot	**1 large** (160g/5³/₄oz)	**7**
Beetroot	**2 small**	**5**
Boiled potato	*3 small (60g/2¹/₈oz)*	*5*
Sweet potato	*1 (120g/4¹/₄oz)*	*10*
Baked potato	*1 (120g/4¹/₄oz)*	*10*
French fries	*10 fries*	*10*

GRAINS, BREADS, CEREALS

Quinoa (cooked)	**65g/2¹/₄oz (²/₃ cup)**	**5**
Pearl Barley (cooked)	**75g/(2³/₄oz)**	**5**
Brown basmati rice (cooked)	**1 small serving (70g/(2¹/₂oz)**	**5**
White rice (cooked)	*¹/₂ serving (65g/2¹/₄oz)*	*10*
Couscous (soaked)	*¹/₂ serving (65g/2¹/₄oz)*	*10*
Rough oatcakes	**2–3 oatcakes**	**5**
Pumpernickel-style rye bread	**1 thin slice**	**5**
Wholemeal bread	**1 thin slice**	**5**
Bagel	**¹/₄ bagel**	**5**
Puffed rice cakes	**1 rice cake**	**5**
White pasta	*1 small serving (75g/2³/₄oz)*	*10*

BEANS AND LENTILS

Soya beans	**3¹/₂ cans**	**5**
Pinto beans	**1 can**	**5**
Lentils	**³/₄ can**	**7**
Kidney beans	**¹/₂ can**	**7**
Chickpeas	**¹/₃ can**	**7**
Baked beans	**¹/₃ can**	**7**

For a complete list of foods and their GL scores, log on to www.holforddiet.com.

What to eat for breakfast

First of all, don't skip breakfast. It's your most important meal of the day. When you wake up after a night's sleep, your blood sugar will be low because you haven't eaten for many hours, therefore it's important to refuel with a good breakfast that will raise your energy levels and your mood. Even if you don't feel particularly hungry, eating a small amount of a low-GL breakfast will prevent you getting hungrier later in the morning – when you're more likely to opt for an unhealthy option such as coffee and a croissant.

Many people make the fatal mistake of not eating anything for breakfast and instead prop themselves up with liquid stimulants (coffee or tea) or nicotine. However, as your blood sugar level dips lower and lower, you're likely to buckle under the strain and end up bingeing out on high-GL foods, such as a piece of toast or a croissant. Sounds familiar?

That's why you must eat breakfast. The only questions are what and how much? There are three fundamental breakfasts that give you the right balance of both carbohydrate and protein. These are:

Carbohydrates		Protein
Cereal or fruit	plus	seeds/yoghurt/milk
Bread or toast	plus	egg
Bread or toast	plus	fish (such as kippers or smoked salmon)

The next question is which type of cereal, fruit or toast should you have and how much? Let's kick off with the cereal-based breakfasts, sweetened with fruit rather than sugar.

The best cereal-based breakfasts

A good cereal-based breakfast needs to include a low-GL cereal, a low-GL fruit as a sweetener, and a source of protein and essential fats, with the goal being no more than 10 GL points.

In the chart overleaf you'll see six cereals and the quantity for each that equals 5 GL points. As you can see, the best 'value' in terms of your appetite are oat flakes, either cooked as porridge or eaten raw, just like you would cornflakes. Basically, you could eat as many as you like, given that one very large bowl (75g) will fill anybody up.

Cereal	5 GL points
Oat flakes	2 servings (75g/2¾oz)
All Bran	1 serving (25g/1oz)
Unsweetened muesli	1 small serving (15g/½oz)
Alpen	½ serving (15g/½oz)
Raisin Bran	⅓ serving (15g/½oz)
Weetabix	1 biscuit (10g/¼oz)
Cornflakes	¼ serving (7g/⅛oz)

Below, you can see six fruits and the quantity you could eat for each to equal 5 GL points:

Fruit	5 GL points
Strawberries	1 large punnet
Pear	1
Grapefruit	1
Apple	1 small
Peach	1 small
Banana	less than ½
Raisins	10

So, your all-time best bet would be to have unsweetened oat flakes with as many strawberries as you could eat. Alternatively, you could have a bowl of All Bran and a grapefruit, or a bowl of unsweetened muesli without raisins in it, with a small grated apple.

As far as protein is concerned, there's some in cow's milk (or in soya milk). Rice milk is quite high in GLs and is best kept to a minimum. Oat milk is a lower GL than rice milk but higher than soya milk. Yoghurt is high in protein, so it is reasonably low in GLs, but it must be unsweetened. So, having a spoonful of yoghurt on your cereal helps to stabilise your blood sugar.

Another source of protein – as well as containing countless vitamins, minerals, essential fats and fibre – are seeds. I recommend you have a tablespoon of ground seeds on your cereal as well. This adds lots of flavour and, by giving yourself the healthy essential fats you need, you won't crave less desirable food sources of fat.

FOR MOOD-BOOSTING WITHOUT LOSING WEIGHT

Remember that if you don't need to lose weight, or once your weight is stabilised, you still need to keep your blood sugar even, so increase your carbs during the day to be no more than 60 GLs.

The best egg-based breakfasts

Although it is true that more than half the calories in an egg come from fat, the kind of fat depends on the type of feed the chicken has been given. Most eggs come from battery chickens. If you knew how unhealthy they were, you probably wouldn't want to eat their eggs, which are high in saturated fat; however, there are some types of eggs that are laid by free-range chickens fed omega-3-rich feed, for example, flaxseeds (Columbus is such a range – it's sold in most big supermarkets). Either these or organic eggs are much better for you. You can have up to seven eggs a week for their mood-boosting properties. However, if you're trying to lose weight, I recommend you have no more than four eggs a week – and only these kinds of eggs. Have either two small eggs, or one large. Poach them, boil them or scramble them, but don't fry them, as the high heat damages the essential fats.

As eggs are pure protein and fat, what carbohydrate can you have with them? If this is your breakfast choice, you can use up your entire 10 GL quota by having any of the following bread servings.

Bread	10 GL points
Oatcakes	4 biscuits
Pumpernickel-style rye bread	2 thin slices
Sourdough rye bread	2 thin slices

Rye wholemeal bread (yeasted)	1 slice
Wheat wholemeal bread (yeasted)	1 slice
White, high-fibre bread (yeasted)	less than 1 slice

As you can see, your best 'value' breads are either oatcakes or Scandinavian-style pumpernickel breads or sourdough rye bread, made without yeast. These are real breads; unlike the light, white, fluffy 'fake' breads we've been conditioned to eat by adding flavour enhancers, sugar and numerous chemicals. So, do try them, as they are more sustaining for your appetite, even though you might find the flavours unusual to begin with. Because these breads are naturally high in fibre and cooked slowly (in the case of pumpernickel) or risen without adding yeast (in the case of sourdough) their GL score is lower.

Breads for fish breakfasts

If you're having a fish breakfast, include the same amount of bread as listed for the egg-based breakfasts.

What to eat for snacks

Individuals with sugar sensitivity are likely to reach for snack foods to compensate for changes in blood sugar levels and hormonal responses, but most commercial snacks are incredibly high in sugar or fat. A Mars Bar, for example, is almost two-thirds sugar with the rest being mainly fat, while even some so-called 'muesli' bars are deceptively unhealthy, made with refined sugar, dates and raisins (which are also high in sugar), and large quantities of hydrogenated fat.

However, research clearly shows that 'grazing' (eating little and often) is healthier for you than 'gorging' (having one or two big meals in the day).[219] One advantage is that it keeps your blood sugar level even. For this reason I recommend you have a mid-morning and a mid-afternoon snack. The ideal snack is one that provides no more than 5 GL points as well as some protein. The simplest snack food is fruit. Let's see what you'd need to eat to stay within 5 GL points for your snack.

Fruit	5 GL points
Strawberries	1 large punnet
Plums	4
Cherries	1 small punnet
Pear	1
Grapefruit	1
Orange	1
Apple	1 small (to fit into the palm of your hand)
Peach	1 small
Melon/watermelon	1 slice

Berries, plums and cherries are your best 'value' fruit snacks. Berries include raspberries, blueberries, blackberries, and any others that you can get your hands on in season. They are low in GL because the principal type of sugar they contain is called xylose. This has about half the GL of fructose, the principal sugar in apples and pears. This again, is about half the GL of glucose or dextrose, the principal sugar in grapes, dates and bananas. You can further lower the glycemic load of these fruits by eating them with five almonds or two teaspoons of pumpkin seeds, both of which are high in protein.

Another snack option would be some kind of bread with a protein-based spread. Cottage cheese, humous or nut butters such as peanut, almond or cashew, are good examples. Humous is very low in GL and tastes great with oatcakes or rye bread, or with a raw carrot (a large carrot is still less than 5 GLs). If you choose humous or a nut butter without added sugar, plus a slice of the bread servings described above, this will give you the right mix of low-GL carbohydrate with protein to keep your blood sugar level even.

So here is a selection of 5 GL snacks to choose from:

- A piece of fruit, plus five almonds or two teaspoons of pumpkin seeds.
- A thin slice of wholemeal bread, pumpernickel-style rye bread or sourdough, or two oatcakes, and half a small tub of cottage cheese (150g/5½oz).
- A piece of bread/two oatcakes and half a small tub of humous (150g/5½oz).

- A piece of bread/two oatcakes and peanut butter.
- Crudités (a carrot, pepper, cucumber or celery) and humous.
- Crudités or berries and cottage cheese.
- A small, plain soya or dairy yoghurt (150g/5½oz), no sugar, plus berries.

What to eat for lunch and dinner

The easiest way to get the balance right for your main meals is to imagine your dinner on a plate. Half the plate will consist of very low-GL vegetables. These vegetables, listed overleaf, will not account for any more than 4 GL points.

The perfect diet plate

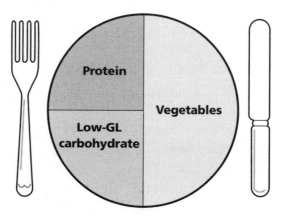

The other half of your plate is divided in two, one for protein-based food, such as meat, fish (or tofu, for example, if you are vegetarian) and the other quarter for more 'starchy' vegetables, accounting for 6–7 GL points. So, a quarter of what's on your plate is protein rich, a quarter is carbohydrate rich and half is made up of very low-GL vegetables. You'll soon get the hang of it. It's very straightforward.

Starchy vegetables

As a rough guide, the serving size of the carbohydrate-rich 'starchy vegetable' food should be more or less the same weight, or size, as the serving of the protein-rich food. If you are eating chicken, which is quite dense and heavy, with rice, which is quite light, the serving size of rice will be somewhat larger than the piece of chicken for each to be roughly the same weight.

Let's take a look at the quantity of different starchy vegetables you can eat to keep within 10 GL points per meal, leaving 3 GL points for the 'unlimited vegetables' that make up half your plate.

Starchy vegetables	7 GL points
Pumpkin/squash	1 large serving (185g/6½oz)
Carrot	1 large (160g/5¾oz)
Swede	1 large serving (150g/5½oz)
Quinoa	1 large serving (120g/4¼oz)
Beetroot	1 large serving (110g/3¾oz)
Cornmeal	1 serving (115g/4oz)
Pearl barley	1 small serving (95g/3¼oz)
Wholemeal pasta	½ serving (85g/3oz)
White pasta	½ serving (65g/2¼oz)
Brown rice	1 small serving (70g/2½oz)
White rice	⅓ serving (45g/1½oz)
Couscous	⅓ serving (45g/1½oz)
Broad beans	1 serving (30g/1oz)
Sweet corn	½ cob (60g/2⅛oz)
Boiled potato	3 small potatoes (75g/2¾oz)
Baked potato	½ (60g/2⅛oz)
French fries	1 tiny portion (45g/1½oz)
Sweet potato	½ (60g/2⅛oz)

As you can see, there are some obvious winners. Wholemeal pasta, for example spaghetti, and brown basmati rice are much better than white pasta and white rice. (There are also some specialist low-GL pastas, called Dreamfield, and strains of low-GL rice, called Maharani rice, available from Totally Nourish – see Resources. These allow you to increase the portion size – and they taste delicious. Another pasta option is Del Ugo's chickpea pasta, available in some supermarkets.) Swede, carrot and squash are much better than potato. Boiled potato is better than baked potato, which is better than French fries.

Beans and lentils

The best foods for balancing your blood sugar and giving the right mix of protein and carbohydrate are beans and lentils. In fact, it's the combination of protein and carbohydrate in beans and lentils that keeps their GL score low. So, any meal containing beans and lentils as both the protein and the carbohydrate source can be quite generous with the portion size because you are getting both protein and carbohydrate from the same food.

However, when you are eating these foods as your source of protein, combine with *half* the serving size of a carbohydrate-rich food, instead of an equal serving. So, for example, if you were making a bean and rice dish, you would have a cup of cooked lentils and half a cup of cooked rice. This is because beans and lentils also contain a significant amount of carbohydrate.

This is how much you can eat, assuming you are not eating another starchy vegetable, to stay within 7 GL points.

Beans and lentils	7 GL points
Soya beans	2 cans
Pinto beans	¾ can
Lentils	¾ can
Baked beans	⅓ can
Butter beans	½ can
Split peas	½ can
Kidney beans	½ can
Chickpeas	⅓ can

Try the Chestnut and Butterbean Soup recipe (see page 205) for an example of an easy recipe that takes minutes and makes a perfect snack or meal with a salad and oatcakes.

Unlimited vegetables

Now it's time to move on to the other half of your plate. This is made up of what I call the 'unlimited vegetables'. Of course, there are limits even to vegetable choices, but these particular vegetables are those for which a serving is less than 2 GL points. A serving, in this context, is quite small – 115g (4oz) peas or 100g (3½oz) broccoli, for example. I want you to eat two servings of unlimited vegetables, one serving of 'starchy' vegetables and one serving of protein-based food – and feel full at the end of every meal.

Asparagus	Cucumber	Peas
Aubergine	Endive	Peppers
Beansprouts	Fennel	Radish
Broccoli	Garlic	Rocket
Brussels sprouts	Kale	Runner beans
Cabbage	Lettuce	Spinach
Cauliflower	Mangetouts	Spring onions
Celery	Mushrooms	Tomato
Courgette	Onions	Watercress

Desserts and drinks

Provided the basic foods you choose are low-GL you can enjoy occasional desserts and an alcoholic drink without suffering from mood swings connected to blood sugar dips and without gaining weight or losing energy. If you wish to lose weight, you can have an additional 5 GLs for drinks or snacks. If weight loss isn't an issue, you don't have to be quite so strict. This means, as part of the weight-loss diet, you could have a dessert on Monday, a glass of wine on Tuesday, a drink and a dessert on Wednesday, but neither on Thursday. That's as hard as it gets. (In my books, *The Low-GL Diet Bible* and *The Holford Low-GL Diet Cookbook*, and *Food GLorious Food*, co-authored with Fiona McDonald Joyce, we have created all kinds of low-GL desserts.)

To keep your blood sugar under control you need to be really careful about what you drink. Estimates suggest that two thirds of the increase in sugar in our modern diets come from drinks – including natural fruit juices. It's a lot easier to drink a glass of grape juice, for example, than to eat a whole bunch of grapes. At the other end of the scale a 2 litre (3½ pint) bottle of cola has roughly 45 teaspoonfuls of sugar in it! The chart below shows you what you can drink for 5 GLs.

Drink	5 GLS
Tomato juice	1 pint
Carrot juice	1 small glass
Grapefruit juice, unsweetened	1 small glass
CherryActive concentrate*	1 small glass, diluted 50:50 with water
Apple juice, unsweetened	1 small glass, diluted 50:50 with water
Orange juice, unsweetened	1 small glass, diluted 50:50 with water; or the juice of 1 orange
Pineapple juice	½ small glass, diluted 50:50 with water
Cranberry juice drink	½ small glass, diluted 50:50 with water
Grape juice	2.5cm (1 inch) of liquid!

*See Resources for details.

A good rule of thumb is to have no more than one glass of juice a day, diluting it as you need to in order to have no more than 5 GLs a day. So have, say, either a glass of carrot juice, or a diluted apple juice or cherry concentrate.

Remember, bananas and grapes are fast releasing, apples and pears medium releasing (predominantly fructose) whereas cherries, berries and plums are slow releasing (predominantly xylose). So, if you pick a smoothie, don't go for one where the top two ingredients are bananas and grape juice. Most of all, stay away from all fizzy, sweetened, caffeinated drinks and sugar-sweetened cordials.

What about alcohol?

Whole books have been written extolling the merits and dangers of alcohol. In our 100% Health Survey, drinking a small amount of alcohol had no negative effect in relation to mood or energy, but that means a small glass of wine, and not every day. From a blood sugar point of view, small amounts of 'dry' drinks such as dry wine or champagne, or spirits such as a whisky, are not a big issue. The mixers, such as tonic and cola are more of a problem, however. Beer has a higher GL value so, again, it is better to go for dry lagers. My advice is to have an occasional, not a daily, drink, perhaps four times a week. If you find you are drinking every day to numb negative feelings, then it's time to face whatever it is that's making you feel bad. See Chapter 16.

Good-mood meals

Here are a few ideas for quick healthy meals.

- Try grilled chicken breasts, seasoned with garlic and herbs, or lay a fillet of fish over sliced peppers and an onion in a lightly oiled shallow ovenproof dish, brush with oil and toss with a little rosemary, then grill.

- Stir-fry chicken strips before adding vegetables or add cubed fish to the last few minutes of a vegetable stir-fry.

- Cooked fish, such as smoked mackerel, can be flaked into large pieces and served in a mixed salad with a drizzle of dressing. Top an omelette with smoked salmon strips and put under the grill to heat through.

- If you enjoy pasta, make a simple sauce by adding a can of cannellini beans to a home-made tomato sauce and flavour it with chopped coriander or parsley.

- Try quinoa, for a change, to serve with sauce-based dishes or curries. Accompany dishes with brown basmati rice or mashed sweet potato or butternut squash and steamed vegetables.

- Soups are always popular and can be very quick to make with a variety of pulses and vegetables. Red lentils take just 20 minutes to cook and can be made into a tasty soup with onion, celery, a can of tomatoes, stock and a good pinch of chilli flakes.

HEALTHY COOKING TECHNIQUES

Steaming is the best way to cook leafy vegetables as it retains all the nutrients. Avoid over-cooking – vegetables are healthiest and taste best when cooked al dente, that's just tender with a bit of bite.

Steam-frying is a good way to cook vegetables and poultry without using oil. Add 2 tbsp of liquid to the pan (water, vegetable stock, soy sauce or watered-down pasta sauce). Bring to the boil and then immediately add some vegetables. Cook rapidly for 1–2 minutes, then turn up the heat and add 2 tbsp more of the liquid. Put on a tight-fitting lid, then steam until the vegetables are cooked. If you're cooking poultry, cut into thin strips and add this at the beginning. Make sure it's cooked through before adding the vegetables.

Stir-frying with 1 tbsp oil is also a healthy way to cook vegetables and poultry.

Grilling Brush poultry, meat or fish lightly with oil and avoid over-browning.

Mood-boosting recipes

Although you can obviously put together your own meals and recipes, choosing good-mood foods, here's a few of my favourite mood-boosting recipes, most of which were created by my kitchen wizard, Fiona McDonald Joyce.

Breakfasts

Low-carb Muesli Stir together 100g (3½oz) whole oat flakes, 50g (1¾oz) ground almonds, 2 tbsp pumpkin seeds, 2 tbsp macadamia nuts, roughly chopped, 2 tbsp sunflower seeds and 2 tsp xylitol (a low-GL sugar alternative) and mix with milk or soya milk. Serves 2

Low-GL Granola Heat 1 tbsp coconut oil or olive oil in a frying pan and add 1 tbsp xylitol and 50g (1¾oz) whole oat flakes. Stir for 3 minutes or until they start to go golden and crisp up slightly. Add 1 tbsp flaked almonds and 1 tbsp macadamia nuts, roughly chopped. Cook for 2 minutes. Remove from the heat and stir in 1 tbsp pumpkin seeds or ground chia seeds and 1 tbsp ground almonds. Serves 2

Smoked Salmon and Chive Scrambled Eggs Beat 4 medium eggs with ground black pepper in a bowl. Heat 2 tsp coconut oil or olive oil in a small pan over gentle heat and pour in the egg. Slowly stir with a wooden spoon to scramble the eggs. Remove the pan from the heat when the eggs are almost set, but still moist. Sprinkle with 2 tsp chopped fresh chives and serve with 75g (2¾oz) smoked salmon. Serves 2

Light lunches

Walnut and Three Bean Salad Mix together 400g (14oz) can mixed beans, a handful of roughly chopped walnuts; ½ cubed apple, 2 tsp chopped fresh flat-leaf parsley or chives, 1 tbsp olive oil, 1 tbsp walnut oil or olive oil, the juice of ½ lemon, 1 finely chopped celery stick, salt and ground black pepper. Serve with mixed salad leaves. Serves 2

Quinoa Tabouleh Put 140g (5oz) quinoa into a pan and add vegetable bouillon powder made up into a liquid to double the quantity of quinoa. Bring to the boil and simmer for 15 minutes or until the liquid is absorbed and the grains are fluffy. Transfer to a bowl and leave to cool. Mix in ¼ cucumber, sliced lengthways into quarters then sliced horizontally; 2 good handfuls of cherry tomatoes, quartered; 4 finely sliced spring onions; a handful of fresh flat-leaf parsley, finely chopped; 1½ tbsp olive oil; 1 tbsp lemon juice; 2 tsp balsamic vineger, or to taste; and salt and ground black pepper. Chill for an hour before serving. Serves 2

Chestnut and Butterbean Soup Put 200g (7oz) cooked and peeled chestnuts (vacuum-packed or canned) into a large pan and add 400g (14oz) can butter beans, 1 chopped onion, 1 chopped carrot, 2 thyme sprigs, 1.2 litres (2 pints) vegetable bouillon or stock and ground black pepper. Bring to the boil and simmer for 35 minutes. Purée until smooth. Serves 4

Smoked Salmon Paté Put 200g (7oz) smoked salmon trimmings into a food processor or blender and add 200g (7oz) canned cannellini beans, the juice of ½ lemon, 1 tbsp chopped fresh parsley, 1 tbsp chopped fresh dill, salt and ground black pepper. Whiz until smooth, adding a drizzle of water or olive oil if necessary. Chill before serving. Serves 2

Fish in an Oriental-style Broth Put 150ml (5fl oz/¼ pint) vegetable bouillon into a wok or large pan and add 2 tbsp mirin, 2 tbsp tamari or soy sauce, 1 small chunk of root ginger, sliced, 2 crushed garlic cloves and 2 lemon slices. Bring to the boil. Add 2 small fish fillets (haddock or cod), and cook for 5–10 minutes or until the flesh turns opaque and flakes easily. Lift out of the pan and remove the skin. Divide the fish between two soup bowls, cover and keep warm. Add the following vegetables to the broth at 30-second intervals, cooking until al dente: 55g (2oz) broccoli florets, 55g (2oz) carrots, coarsely grated; 55g (2oz) pak choi, finely shredded; 4 thinly sliced spring onions. Remove the vegetables and add to the bowls. Boil the broth for 30 seconds, then remove the ginger and lemon. Stir in ½ tsp sesame oil, ladle over the fish and vegetables. Serves 2

Main meals

Tuna Steak with Black-eyed Bean Salsa In a bowl, mix together 2 tomatoes, deseeded and chopped; 400g (14oz) can black-eyed beans; 1 finely chopped red pepper; 1 mild red chilli, deseeded and finely chopped; 2 crushed garlic cloves; the juice of 2 limes; 2 tsp olive oil; 2 tsp sesame oil; 2 tbsp roughly chopped fresh coriander; and salt and ground black pepper. Set aside. Heat 1 tbsp olive oil in a frying pan. When hot add 2 small tuna steaks. Press firmly into the pan to sear. Turn and sear the other side. Reduce the heat and cook for 1–3 minutes until the flesh flakes easily. Serve with the salsa. Serves 2

Sticky Mustard Salmon Fillets In a bowl, whisk the juice and grated rind of ½ orange with 1 tsp clear honey and 1 tsp wholegrain mustard. Put 2 small skinless and boneless salmon fillets into a shallow dish and pour over the orange mixture. Marinate in the fridge for 30–60 minutes. Preheat the oven to 180°C/350°F/Gas 4. Bake the salmon for 20–25 minutes. Serve with steamed or stir-fried spinach and red peppers, and boiled baby new potatoes or brown basmati rice. Serves 2

Anchovy and Tomato Pasta Put 4 tbsp good-quality tomato-based pasta sauce from a jar into a pan and add 1 tbsp water, 2 tbsp pitted black olives and 2 handfuls of cherry tomatoes, halved. Simmer until the tomatoes start to soften. Stir in 50g (1¾oz) fresh anchovy fillets (from the deli), chopped, and season well with ground black pepper. Serve over wholemeal pasta. Serves 2

Puy Lentils with Porcini Mushrooms and Thyme Soak 25g (1oz) dried porcini mushrooms for 30 minutes in warm water, then drain, reserving the liquor. Cook 200g (7oz) dried Puy lentils according to the pack instructions, using the liquor from the soaked mushrooms and water. Heat 1 tbsp mild olive oil in a small frying pan and cook 2 crushed garlic cloves, 1 diced red onion, 1 finely chopped celery stick, and 2 finely chopped leeks for 2 minutes. Cover and cook over a low heat for a further 5 minutes to soften. Stir the lentils into the pan with the soaked mushrooms and 50g (2oz) walnut pieces, roughly chopped. Add 1 tbsp fresh thyme, and salt and ground black pepper. Serves 2

Chickpea Curry Heat 2 tsp olive oil in a large frying pan and fry 2 crushed garlic cloves for 1 minute. Add 1 large chopped onion, 1 tsp cumin, ½ tsp turmeric, ½ tsp medium curry powder and 1 tsp ground ginger, and cook for 2 minutes. Add 1 finely chopped celery stick and 1 chopped medium carrot. Measure 600ml (20fl oz/1 pint) vegetable stock in a jug then take 2 tbsp stock and add to the pan. Cover and cook gently for 2 minutes. Add 400g (14oz) can chickpeas, 2 tbsp tomato purée and a little salt. Stir in the remaining stock. Bring to the boil and simmer uncovered for 30 minutes, or until the vegetables are tender. Serves 2

Desserts

Baked Apple with Spiced Blackberry Stuffing Preheat the oven to 180°C/350°F/Gas 4. In a small bowl, mix ¼ tsp cinnamon, 2 tsp xylitol and 2 tbsp blackberries together. Put 2 cored cooking apples in an ovenproof dish and stuff with the mixture. Bake for 35–40 minutes, or until soft right through without collapsing. Serves 2

Blueberry Oat Pancakes Put 50g (1¾oz) cornflour into a blender jug and add 50g (1¾oz) oat flour, 35g (1¼oz) xylitol, 200ml (7fl oz/⅓ pint) skimmed milk, soya milk or nut milk, 2½ tbsp water and 1 medium egg. Whiz until smooth. Heat 1 tsp coconut oil or butter in a frying pan and tip to coat the whole surface. Spoon in a quarter of the batter and tip the pan to spread it evenly over the base. Cook for 30–45 seconds, or until starting to firm on the top, then turn over and cook the other side until pale golden. Remove from the pan and keep warm while you make the others. Put 4 tbsp blueberries in a small pan with 2 tsp xylitol, 1 tbsp water and 1 tsp lemon juice. Heat gently until the berries start to burst. Spoon a little into the middle of each pancake and fold up. Serves 4

Carrot and Walnut Cake Preheat the oven to 180°C/350°F/Gas 4. Grease and line a 10cm (4 inch) mini-cake tin with baking parchment. In a bowl, cream together 50g (1¾oz) coconut oil or butter (at room temperature) and 50g (1¾oz) xylitol until soft and smooth. Stir in 50g (1¾oz) organic soya flour, ¼ tsp baking powder and 50g (1¾oz) ground walnuts. Mix in 50g (1¾oz) chopped walnuts and 1 finely grated medium carrot, then stir in 2 medium eggs. Spoon into the tin and bake for 35 minutes or until the top is risen and golden. Cover the top with foil and bake for a further 20 minutes or until a skewer inserted into the centre comes out clean. Cool for 15 minutes in the tin, then turn out and cool completely. In a bowl, mix 50g (1¾oz) low-fat cream cheese with ½ tsp vanilla extract and 1 tsp xylitol. Spread over the top of the cake. Serves 4

Chapter 18

MOOD-BOOSTING SUPPLEMENTS

The purpose of nutrient supplementation is to ensure that your body and brain have 24-hour access to all the nutrients they need to be in optimal health. Many essential nutrients are inadequately supplied, not only in the average 21st-century diet but also in those who think that they eat a well-balanced diet; for example, most people do not achieve optimal levels of vitamins B_{12}, C and D nor omega-3 fats, to name a few.

However, there is one fundamental truth that we have seen countless examples of in Part 2, and that is when your system is out of balance it takes a much higher intake of nutrients to bring it back. An optimal level of chromium, for example, is around 50mcg a day, but the amount needed if you suffer from atypical depression is around 500mcg. Similarly, a good daily intake of vitamin B_{12} is around 10mcg, but if you have marginal deficiency you may require 500mcg to correct this. (This big difference is largely because B_{12} is difficult to absorb, so you need to swallow a *lot* more to absorb a *little* more.)

This creates two levels of 'need': the intake of nutrients you need to optimise your health on a daily basis – which I call the 'basics' – and the intake you need to bring your system back into balance, which I call the 'extras'. Your need for extra supplements is guided by your responses to the symptom-based questionnaires you took in Part 2 and any blood tests that you have had. You will not need to take the extras for long, as the body can generally correct biochemical imbalances within six months, and sometimes quicker. But, once you are feeling better, and your questionnaire scores have become optimal, it is best to continue with the extras for a month before stopping that supplement.

All these supplements are available from health-food stores or via the Internet. It is best to choose reliable companies with a track record of manufacturing good-quality products. The Resources section on supplements and suppliers gives you examples of recommended supplements and companies to help you find what you need.

The basics

My basics for a good supplement programme are based on my estimates of what is optimal as a total intake, minus what you can achieve from a reasonably healthy diet. The difference is what you supplement. The optimal intake for a nutrient is called the ODA (optimal daily allowance) and you can see the ODA for each nutrient, versus what we can achieve from our diet, on www.patrickholford.com/oda.

The easiest way to achieve the difference – that is the levels of nutrients worth supplementing every day – is to take three daily supplements:

1 An 'optimum nutrition' multivitamin and mineral.

2 Extra vitamin C, including other synergistic immune-boosting nutrients.

3 An essential omega-3 and -6 supplement.

I take these every day and recommend that you do the same. But how do you know which formulations to choose?

The best multis

The packaging on any decent multivitamin and mineral will tell you to take two a day, preferably one with breakfast and one with lunch; firstly because you cannot get enough of all the nutrients in one pill, and secondly because the water-soluble vitamins B and C are in and out of your body in four to six hours, so you get twice the benefit taking them twice a day.

Many multivitamins skimp on the minerals. A hallmark of a good one is that it provides at least 100mg of magnesium, 10mg of zinc plus 25mcg of selenium and chromium. Another hallmark is its vitamin D content. You need at least 10mcg, ideally 15mcg a day. Also, make sure there are enough B vitamins; for example, you need 10mcg of B_{12} and 20mg of B_6. Supplements that provide all these 'optimal' levels are more expensive than basic RDA-based multivitamins because they contain much higher levels of nutrients. That's because the RDA for B_{12} is 1mcg and for B_6 it's 2mg – a tenth of the optimal level.

The best vitamin C supplements

The form of vitamin C itself doesn't make as much difference as people make out. Ascorbic acid, ascorbate, 'ester' C – they all work. But there are other nutrients and herbs that support health and immunity. These include zinc, black elderberry extracts, anthocyanidins (for example in bilberry), ginger, echinacea and cat's claw. (In the UK these last two are classified as medicinal herbs and can't be added to supplements, but they can be taken on their own.) So, a vitamin C supplement that also contains these synergistic ingredients gives you more bang for your buck. Ideally, you want something like 2,000mg of vitamin C in total a day, but you will achieve 200mg of this if you eat six or more servings of the right fruit and vegetables a day. So that leaves 1,800mg to supplement – or 900mg twice a day. That's a good level for general health maintenance and health insurance.

The best essential-fat supplements

The most potent forms of omega-3 are called EPA, DPA and DHA. These are found in oily fish. The most potent omega-6 is called GLA. This is found in borage and evening primrose oil. We need more omega-3, and are also more deficient in it, so you want at least ten times more omega-3 than -6. (Add up the total EPA, DPA and DHA in a supplement and divide by the total GLA. This figure should be over 10.) In all you are looking for at least 600mg of combined EPA, DPA and DHA a day for general health maintenance.

The extras for improved mood

The following supplements are well worth trying if you scored high on the questionnaires in Part 2 or blood tests have confirmed you have imbalances. There's no harm, as such, in doing all of them but it might be a bit of overkill; however, don't double up on doses. For example, if you are a candidate for 5-HTP in the serotonin check and the sleep check – each recommending 100mg a day – don't add them together and take 200mg a day; however, if any nutrient does come up twice, there's a good chance that this nutrient will be important for you. If you scored high on three or more factors, then focus on your top three 'extras'.

Most of these extra supplements work within 7 to 30 days, so you should be able to get a pretty quick indication if they are going to help you. If they don't, try something else. A good way to gauge how they are working for you is to set yourself a monthly supplement programme, and stick to it as best you can. If you skip one day out of six, that's not the end of the world, but ideally you want to take supplements twice a day, every day. Then, at the end of the month, rescore yourself on the mood questionnaire on page 7.

Each of the extras listed relates to a chapter in part 2.

Chromium

Check out chromium if you are tired and craving; that is, if you scored high on the blood sugar check in Chapter 7, page 58, and/or you have one or more of the symptoms of atypical depression described on page 64.

Buy a supplement of either chromium picolinate or polynicotinate 200mcg and take two in the morning and one at midday or at lunchtime. It doesn't matter if you take it with or without food. If you get a positive effect on your mood, energy and possibly on food cravings within a week, keep taking it for another week, then lower the dose to one in the morning and one at midday. If the results aren't then as positive, go back to three a day. If this feels right, take the supplement for at least a week. Then try taking one a day, in the morning. If this doesn't work, go back to two a day. After two months, see what happens if you stop.

Your basic multivitamin needs to provide at least 30mcg of chromium. Some people benefit from a higher maintenance dose of 200mcg. Find out what works for you. The toxic level of chromium is 10,000mcg, so you are not going to overdose on it!

Tyrosine

Take tyrosine if you suspect you have an underactive thyroid, if you scored high on the thyroid check in Chapter 8, page 69, or you have had a blood test that determined that your thyroid is underactive. Supplement the extra tyrosine with iodine, selenium and zinc.

L-tyrosine, the natural form of this amino acid, is available in supplements of 500mg. I recommend supplementing 500mg twice a day, morning and afternoon with a carbohydrate snack, ideally away from, or before, a main meal. You can take twice this amount; for example, if you have an underactive thyroid.

Since the enzymes that convert tyrosine into thyroxine are iodine, zinc and selenium-dependent, it's important you also supplement these. A good multivitamin–mineral supplement should provide 30mcg of selenium and 30mcg of iodine plus 10mg of zinc. That's a good starting point, but you can easily double these amounts by taking one kelp tablet (the richest source of iodine) and an additional 100mcg of selenium and 10mg of zinc for extra thyroid support. Seafood is also a rich source of selenium.

Probiotics, glutamine and digestive enzymes

If you scored high on the food sensitivity check in Chapter 9, page 86 or have digestive problems, tune up your digestion with probiotics, glutamine and digestive enzymes. Try supplementing a combination of probiotics (providing both *Lactobacillus acidophilus* and bifidobacteria – at least 1 billion viable organisms) with glutamine and digestive enzymes for a month to give your digestive system a tune-up, as well as identifying and eliminating any foods you may be allergic to.

Omega-3

If you scored high on the essential fat check in Chapter 10, page 93, increase your omega-3s. Supplement twice daily a capsule of essential omega-3 and -6, providing around 250mg of EPA or EPA+DPA. Supplement an additional EPA-rich omega-3 fish oil capsule providing at least 300mg of EPA when you are feeling low. Take this with lunch or dinner so that, together with the basic essential omegas, you are getting some omega-3 fats three times a day. That gives you a total of about 500mg of EPA, plus a further 500mg from eating oily fish three times a week. If you don't eat fish, take two EPA-rich fish oil capsules a day.

Amino acids

If you scored high on the serotonin check in Chapter 11, page 104, add amino acids. Include 100mg of 5-HTP in your daily supplement programme. You need a basic intake of B vitamins (B_6, B_{12} and folic acid, plus niacin – B_3), zinc and magnesium to maximise the conversion of 5-HTP to serotonin, but these will be provided by the basic high-potency multivitamin–mineral. Take 5-HTP with a carbohydrate snack such as some fruit, away from meals or 15 minutes before a meal. You can take twice this amount, 100mg twice a day, morning and afternoon, if you are not on anti-depressants and you don't respond to 100mg.

If you also scored high on the tyrosine check on page 117 you should also take 1,000mg of tyrosine. L-tyrosine, the natural form of this amino acid, is available in supplements of 500mg. I recommend supplementing 500mg twice a day, morning and evening, ideally away from or before a main meal, with a carbohydrate snack. Some formulas provide both 5-HTP and tyrosine (see Resources).

If you live in a country where you can buy SAMe, try taking 400mg a day (200mg twice a day on an empty stomach) for a couple of days, then increase the dose to 400mg twice a day. If you experience any nausea or stomach ache, lower the dose. Be careful with SAMe if you are prone to manic states or phases; consult your doctor beforehand.

Chill-out supplements

If you scored high on the sleep check in Chapter 12, page 126, add 100mg of 5-HTP an hour before bed and make sure you are getting at least 300mg of magnesium a day. A good multivitamin–mineral should provide 100–200mg, so make up the difference with a magnesium supplement in the evening. Some supplements provide combinations of tryptophan, 5-HTP, magnesium and the GABA precursors – taurine and glutamine – plus herbs such as hops, passionflower and valerian. These are preferable and often work out cheaper. If you live in a country where you can buy GABA supplements, take 500mg one hour before bed, but don't combine with valerian. All of these are best taken on an empty stomach or with a carbohydrate snack.

B vitamins

Although a good multivitamin should provide 20mg of B_6, 10mcg of B_{12} and 200mcg of folic acid, if you scored high on the methyl IQ check in Chapter 13, page 144, and have had your homocysteine level checked and found it to be high, you are going to need increased B vitamins to bring your homocysteine level back to normal. See the chart on page 146 to work out the ideal supplemental intake of these homocysteine-lowering B vitamins depending on your particular level. These levels are achieved by supplementing 1–3 methyl nutrient complexes (see Resources, Supplements and Suppliers). Take these for two to three months then recheck your homocysteine level and adjust your dosage accordingly. With the right diet and supplements, most people achieve an optimal homocysteine level within three to six months and can then maintain it with the supplemental basics listed above. Those with genetically inherited poor methylation may need to take a methyl nutrient complex on an ongoing basis.

Vitamin D

If you live above 40 degrees latitude, which includes most of Europe, you will not get enough vitamin D all year round. Ensure you get sufficient vitamin D from spring to early autumn by eating oily fish three times a week and six eggs a week. Also, expose your arms and face for at least 30 minutes a day and take a multivitamin–mineral that provides 15mcg of vitamin D. During the winter, however, this may not be enough. If you feel low in the winter months, supplement an extra 25mcg (or 1,000iu) vitamin D_3 (cholecalciferol) – the kind found in fish. If you are vegetarian, take vitamin D_2 (ergocalciferol), although the D_3 is best.

Are there any dangers?

None of these nutrients, within the dose range given, are dangerous. Some people get mild nausea taking 5-HTP; if this happens to you, lower the dose. Don't take very high levels of folic acid if you don't have a raised homocysteine level. Exceedingly high levels of omega oils may give some people oily skin. If this happens to you, take less.

Supplements are not addictive and do not give rebound withdrawal effects when stopped. They don't store in your body, with the exception of vitamin D, therefore there is no accumulated toxicity issues. There is no logic in taking them for a few weeks and then having a few weeks' break. For best results take them every day, twice a day. That way your brain cells and enzymes have an available supply of the optimal level of nutrients every second of every day.

What if you are taking medication?

Ideally, it is best to discuss any supplements with your doctor if you are taking medication but, sadly, doctors are not trained in nutritional medicine and may have an uninformed bias against it, so you may not get an informed opinion.

I would not recommend taking 5-HTP with antidepressants, although some switched-on psychiatrists give 5-HTP when a person is being weaned off antidepressants, to minimise the withdrawal effects. Don't take GABA with a sleeping pill or tranquilliser. Again, some psychiatrists give GABA during the process of weaning people off sleeping pills and tranquillisers. If you are withdrawing from medication and would like some guidance on nutritional support, read my book *How to Quit Without Feeling S**t*. At the Brain Bio Centre we have a team of psychiatrists and nutritional therapists who can help those who wish to come off drugs, perhaps due to side-effects, by pursuing a nutritional approach instead (see Resources).

What if you are pregnant or breastfeeding?

There is no evidence that any of these nutrients are harmful, or likely to be harmful, during either pregnancy or breastfeeding, to either you or your baby; however, since it is unlikely that these nutrients have been specifically tested on pregnant or breastfeeding women, many supplement companies put a caution on their label. It is likely, however, that some level of nutrients in your bloodstream pass through to the baby in breast milk. This is, of course, an advantage of breastfeeding. Bear in mind, however, that if you are supplementing amino acids, such as 5-HTP or tyrosine, these too may get through. Therefore it is worth being a bit more cautious, perhaps starting with the lower dose-range given, if you are pregnant or breastfeeding.

How long do I keep taking supplements?

The 'basic' supplements shown on page 210 are ideal for anyone to take every day for ever. These kinds of levels, together with a good diet, are the best way to ensure your mental and physical health. The 'extras' are additional supplements to take as long as you need them. If you take any of these and then find your mood, energy and emotional balance have all stabilised, my advice is to keep taking them for an additional one to two months, then experiment with removing the extras, one by one, noticing any return of symptoms. You can also rescore yourself on the various questionnaires, which will give you another yardstick regarding your level of need.

SEEKING NUTRITIONAL SUPPORT

If you feel that you need additional guidance in using supplements, or would prefer one-to-one help, there are nutritional therapists around the UK and in other countries that are trained in the kind of therapies discussed in this book. To find one near you, go to my website (www.patrickholford.com) and within the 'Advice' section you'll see 'Find a Nutritionist' which gives you access to a directory of my recommended nutritional therapists. If you live near Richmond on the south-west of London, or can travel there, our Brain Bio Centre has a dedicated team of highly experienced psychiatrists and nutritional therapists to help you. They also have access to the best biochemical tests for exploring some of the possibilities discussed in Part 2. For further details see Resources.

Most people who visit the clinic start to feel better within the first month, and the supplements prescribed depend on the individual's unique biochemical imbalances. It also requires some effort in terms of controlling your diet. But we continue

CONTINUED...

---

to have frequent reports of major transformations in mood in those with both severe and minor depression. Combined with appropriate psychotherapy and psychological support I do believe nutritional therapy, in almost all cases, produces better results than medication, without any of the undesirable side effects.

Wake up to clear eyes

You may be very surprised to discover the real difference that nutritional therapy can make for you. Stephanie Merritt, a journalist for the *Observer*, who describes her journey through depression in her incredibly moving and honest book *The Devil Within*, came to the Brain Bio Centre after trying conventional treatment with medication. Although the medication was quite effective, she suffered from undesirable side effects. Here is what she found:

CASE STUDY: STEPHANIE

'I had not expected the science to be so sophisticated. My under-informed assumptions about nutrition therapy were that it would be a matter of telling me to drink green tea and eat more oily fish, so that, arriving at the clinic for my first appointment, I had expected to walk away smug in the knowledge that I was already gleaming with nutritional self-righteousness. Instead I was sent off to a lab to have blood, urine and hair samples bagged up and tested for essential mineral and vitamin deficiencies.

'In addition to the lab tests, I had been asked to fill in a highly detailed questionnaire which seemed to cover almost every possible aspect of my mental and physical responses ... Nutrition therapy takes an almost exclusively biochemical approach to mental health (though the centre does recommend talking therapies and regular exercise as supplementary supports) and to a trained nutritionist the answers to all the above questions provide a complete picture of a patient's physical health, which in turn reveals symptoms of underlying deficiencies or allergies that may be affecting mood. Even here the science does not permit

a definitive unravelling of cause and effect – strong emotions such as grief or anger are produced by chemical changes in the brain and create a domino effect of chemical changes in their turn (does a low level of serotonin cause depression, or is it the result?), but the treatment offers a programme which can effectively correct the imbalances underlying the depression, often enabling patients to respond better to therapy or to feel better able to manage their situation.

'I was prescribed an initial daily programme consisting of two high-quality multivitamins, 4g of omega-3 fish oil, an active B_6 and zinc supplement, 2g of vitamin C and 200mg of 5-HTP . . . which increases levels of the amino acid trytophan, a precursor to serotonin.

'About a week after beginning the nutritional supplement programme I had to travel to Edinburgh for work. On my first morning there I woke up in my hotel room and knew immediately that the black mood had lifted . . . It was not a grand sense of elation or joy, just a quiet knowledge that, for the first time in months, I was looking at the world with clear eyes, as it really was. Unspectacular, but not catastrophic. I was no longer being crushed. The unfamiliar room was washed with chilly sunlight and it was startling to recall that this was how it felt to be normal . . . It seemed, to my distinct surprise, that I might be better. I realised that I had not really believed that a cocktail of vitamin supplements bought from a health-food shop could make any noticeable impact on my cladding of hopelessness, but despite my lack of faith, a minor miracle had happened.'

Chapter 19

MAKE EVERY DAY A GOOD DAY

How you start your morning is key to how you will feel for the day that follows. The trick is to start it well, and having a healthy breakfast is probably the most important element, which should be part of your routine every single day. If you wake up not feeling great, a healthy breakfast, plus taking your mood-boosting supplements, will give your system a kick-start. Factor in some vital-energy-generating exercises, such as movement and stretches, or perhaps go for a walk and practise mindfulness. Some people like to listen to an uplifting piece of music as part of their morning routine or do something else that they enjoy. Ideally, take your exercise when you first get up, or after your bath or shower. If your energy is low, have a piece of fruit for a quick pick-me-up. I like to start my day by doing Psychocalisthenics, which is a 16-minute exercise routine that generates vital energy and mindfulness as well as a balanced mood, and it keeps you fit and supple too.

Here are some other tips to keep you feeling good:

Start your day with a big result. Pick one thing that's important for you to do, and do that first rather than doing all the little jobs, while resisting the larger ones.

Don't use sugar to reward yourself or cheer yourself up. Take some chromium instead and make yourself a good, healthy meal or a low-GL snack.

Be careful about alcohol and other numbing substances. If you find yourself using mind-numbing substances on a regular, or daily, basis to avoid uncomfortable feelings, a healthier alternative is to take some action to deal with what is troubling you.

Make time for exercise. I recommend you make an appointment in your diary, just as you would for any other appointment, and make this your time for exercising. Ideally, exercise outdoors. Exercise helps to boost your mood, which increases the feel-good endorphins as well as your serotonin levels. Going for a brisk walk in your local park or in natural surroundings is a great thing to do regularly, but particularly if you feel down or upset. Walk the feelings out. There's something centring about having your feet on the earth. It's your diminutive version of going walkabout.

Generate vital energy. Particularly beneficial are what I call vital-energy-generating exercises such as yoga, t'ai chi and Psychocalisthenics. There's growing evidence that these all help to improve your mood.[220] Fundamental to their practice is a specific pattern of breathing and 'mindfulness' which, as we saw in Chapter 16, has many positive benefits. The practice of these kinds of exercises are 'centring' in the sense that they move you out of becoming stuck in thoughts and feelings into a state of mindful awareness. Exercises like this are designed to generate energy, called *chi* in China. Perhaps the easiest to learn is Psychocalisthenics, which can be practised at home; however, it is also good to have some group practice, and yoga classes are widely available. Once you learn some of the postures, you will also be able to practise yoga at home. See Resources for more details.

Get enough sleep. Sleep is as vital as any nutrient. To help you, take the sleep nutrients listed in the previous chapter, but also make sure your bedroom is good for sleeping. Use soft lighting when you go to bed, perhaps having a warm bath with relaxing essential oils, such as lavender, first. Play the CD *Silence of Peace* (see Resources) quietly. If you can't sleep, read a good book, but not something dark and depressing. If you wake up in the night, put the CD back on. If your mind is wide awake, get up and do something; perhaps read your book, then go back to sleep when you feel tired. Don't lie in bed stressing about not sleeping.

Get enough light. Don't go to bed too late; it's important to wake up early in the morning, ideally not long after the sun comes up. Of course, this depends on the time of year and where you live but, ideally, your curtains should let through sufficient light to help you wake naturally at dawn. In winter, if you need to get up before dawn, buy a dawn alarm. In the early evening, when it gets dark early, expose yourself to more light with full spectrum lighting, a full spectrum reading light or a light box (see Resources). Go outside every day so that you receive some light that is not reaching you through glass, perhaps a walk in the park or to the shops. Make the most of being outdoors in the autumn; that's when your body stores vitamin D for the winter. If you can, get a winter holiday in the sun.

Do what you can to reduce your stress levels. Stress often results from having unfinished business and unrealistic goals. Learn to say no and don't take on something new until you have finished the last task. Don't have unrealistic expectations of yourself.

Respect your feelings. No one feels happy all the time. It is natural to experience sadness, anger and fear, and it is completely healthy to feel depressed when you are processing significant losses in life. Your feelings are there to show you something. The trick is to understand how you can learn from them and how to express them in a healthy way and then move on. If you truly let yourself experience an uncomfortable feeling, it will change. If you resist a feeling, it will persist. Chapter 16 suggests avenues you can explore to help you move through negative emotional states.

Do something you enjoy every day. Make sure you do something that is just for you every day. If you are a busy mum and get little time to yourself, make some time, even if it is only for a short while. I know one mother who parks her car in a wood between school and work and reads for 15 minutes. That's her time. If you enjoy company, take a break and hang out with a friend, or give them a call. We all need social interaction. Go for a walk in a natural environment. Watch a film. Have a massage. Sign up for a course on something you've always wanted to do. It doesn't matter if you are any good at it; it's fun to learn new things.

Remember that every day is a new day and that you don't have to feel trapped in a cycle. You can break that cycle today, and be free from it every day. I sincerely hope that this book leads you to discover the fundamental keys to feeling good, motivated and sufficiently energised to deal with life's ups and downs, to let go and learn from the past, and to create a lifestyle that makes life a joy to live.

Wishing you the best of health and happiness,

Patrick Holford

REFERENCES

Introduction

1   J. C. Fournier, et al., 'Antidepressant drug effects and depression severity', *Journal of the American Medical Association*, 2010;303(1):47–53

2   D. Healey, et al., 'Association between suicide attempts and selective serotonin reuptake inhibitors: Systematic review of randomised controlled trials', *British Medical Journal*, 2005;330:396–404

3   ibid.

Part 1

4   Prescription Cost Analysis England 2008, NHS, The Information Centre – see www.ic.nhs.uk

5   M. Olfson and S. Marcus, 'National patterns in antidepressant medication treatment', *Archives of General Psychiatry*, 2009;66(8):848–56

6   National Institute of Health and Clinical Excellence, Guideline on 'Depression in adults'; see www.nice.org.uk/CG90

7   P. Boyle, et al., 'Effect of a purpose in life on risk of incident Alzheimer disease and mild cognitive impairment in community-dwelling older persons', *Archives of General Psychiatry*, 2010;67(3):304–10

8   R. A. Waterland and R. L. Jirtle, 'Transposable elements: Targets for early nutritional effects on epigenetic gene regulation', *Molecular and Cellular Biology*, 2003;23:5293–300; see also X. Zhu, et al., 'Maternal deprivation-caused behavioral abnormalities in adult rats relate to a non-methylation-regulated D2 receptor levels in the nucleus accumbens', *Behavioural Brain Research*, June 2010;209(2):281–8. Epub 6 February 2010

9   I. Weaver, et al., 'Reversal of maternal programming of stress responses in adult offspring through methyl supplementation: Altering epigenetic marking later in life', *Journal of Neuroscience*, 2005;25:11045–54

10 N. Marini, et al., 'The prevalence of folate-remedial MTHFR enzyme variants in humans', *Proceedings of the National Academy of Science*, 2008;105(23):8055–60

11 M. Olfson and S. Marcus, 'National patterns in antidepressant medication treatment', *Archives of General Psychiatry*, 2009;66(8):848–56

12 J. C. Fournier, et al., 'Antidepressant drug effects and depression severity', *Journal of the American Medical Association*, 2010;303(1):47–53

13   A. Khan, et al., 'Symptom reduction and suicide risk in patients treated with placebo in antidepressant clinical trials: An analysis of the Food and Drug Administration database', *Archives of General Psychiatry*, 2000;57(4):311–17. The total of 5,200 pages of documents examined revealed that not only were the SSRIs no better than the older tricyclic antidepressants but they were not even 10% more effective than placebos, which produced an average of a 30.9% improvement in depression

14   I. Kirsch, 'Antidepressants and the placebo response', *Epidemiological Psychiatry Society*, 2009 October–December;18(4):318–22; see also I. Kirsch and J. Moncrieff, 'Efficacy of antidepressants in adults', *British Medicine Journal*, July 2005;331(7509):155–7

15   J. C. Fournier, et al., 'Antidepressant drug effects and depression severity', *Journal of the American Medical Association*, 2010;303(1):47–53

16   National Institute of Health and Clinical Excellence, Guideline on 'Depression in adults'; see www.nice.org.uk/CG90

17   *The British National Formulary*, published by the BMJ group, is the doctor's guide to drugs. See www.bnf.org

18   L. Watkins, Conference Report, Annual Meeting of the American Psychosomatic Society in Denver, Colorado, 4 March 2006

19   D. Healy, et al., 'Association between suicide attempts and selective serotonin reuptake inhibitors: Systematic review of randomised controlled trials', *British Medical Journal*, 2005;330:396–404

20   Interview with Dr David Healy, *100% Health Newsletter*, September 2004:22, Holford & Associates Ltd

21   M. H. Teicher, et al., 'Emergence of intense suicidal preoccupation during fluoxetine treatment', *American Journal of Psychiatry*, 1990;147:207–10

22   Personal communication with Dr David Healy, reader in psychological medicine at the North Wales Department of Psychological Medicine, Cardiff University, and the leading campaigner on the links between SSRIs and suicide. His main concern was that doctors should be warned of the possibility of suicide among a small section of patients so that they could take appropriate action. Among his evidence for this risk was the fact that even before the drug was licensed in the UK, precisely such a warning had been insisted on by the German licensing authorities in 1988. It read: 'Patients must be sufficiently observed until the effects of the anti-depressive effect sets in. Taking an additional sedative may also be necessary.'

23   Personal communication with Jerome Burne from Dr David Healy. He told how in 2000 the American paper, the *Boston Globe*, having been alerted to the fact that the patent on Prozac was about to expire, had conducted a search of the US patent office to discover if there was a replacement in the pipeline. A new form of Prozac, known as R-fluoxetine, had been patented in 1993 (US patent no 5,708,035). A patent application requires that you state why your new version is

an improvement. So what were the benefits of R-fluoxetine? 'It will not produce several existing side effects, including akathsia, suicidal thoughts and self-mutilation ... one of its [Prozac's] more significant side effects.' Precisely the side effects the company had been denying for a decade

24   *Independent*, 25 February 2005 (www.independent.co.uk/life-style/health-and-families/health-news/dramatic-increase-in-overdoses-linked-to-anti depressants-484704.html)

25   'Dark secrets lurking in the drugs cabinet', *Observer*, 7 November 2004

26   J. Lenzer, 'FDA warns that antidepressants may increase suicidality in adults', *British Medical Journal*, 2005;331:70

27   See *Guardian* article 'Murder, suicide: A bitter aftertaste for the "wonder" depression drug', at www.guardian.co.uk/Archive/Article/0,4273,4201752,00. html

28   'Symptoms following abrupt discontinuation of duloxetine treatment in patients with major depressive disorder', *Journal of Affective Disorders*, 2005;89(1–3):207– 12

29   F. Bogetto, et al., 'Discontinuation syndrome in dysthymic patients treated with selective serotonin reuptake inhibitors: A clinical investigation', *CNS Drugs*, 2002;16(4):273–83

30   H. Macpherson, et al., 'Closing the evidence gap in integrative medicine', *British Medical Journal*, 1 September 2009;339:b3335

31   K. J. Kemper and K. L. Hood, 'Does pharmaceutical advertising affect journal publication about dietary supplements?', *Complementary & Alternative Medicine*, 9 April 2008:8–11

32   K. Suboticanec, et al., 'Vitamin C status in chronic schizophrenia', *Biological Psychiatry*, 1990;28:959–66

33   E. H. Turner, et al., 'Serotonin a la carte: Supplementation with the serotonin precursor 5-hydroxytryptophan', *Pharmacology and Therapeutics*, March 2006;109(3):325–38

34   I. Bjelland, et al., 'Folate, vitamin B_{12}, homocysteine, and the MTHFR 677CT polymorphism in anxiety and depression: The Hordaland Homocysteine Study', *Archives of General Psychiatry*, 2003;60:618–26

35   A. Coppen and J. Bailey, 'Enhancement of the antidepressant action of fluoxetine by folic acid', *Journal of Affective Disorders*, 2000;60:121–30

36   M. J. Taylor, et al., 'Folate for depressive disorders', *Cochrane Database of Systematic Reviews*, 2003;2. Art. No: CD003390. DOI: 10.1002/14651858.CD003390.

37   J. R. Hibbeln, 'Fish consumption and major depression', *Lancet*, 1998; 351(9110):1213

38   V. Bountziouka, et al., 'Long-term fish intake is associated with less severe depressive symptoms among elderly men and women: The MEDIS (MEDiterranean ISlands Elderly) epidemiological study', *Journal of Aging and Health*, September 2009;21(6):864–80

39 J. R. Hibbeln, 'Seafood consumption and homicide mortality: A cross-national ecological analysis', *World Review of Nutrition and Dietetics*, 2001;88:41–6

40 B. Hallahan, et al., 'Omega-3 fatty acid supplementation in patients with recurrent self-harm: Single-centre double-blind randomised controlled trial', *British Journal of Psychiatry*, 2007 Feb;190:118–22

41 M. E. Virkkunen, et al., 'Plasma phospholipid essential fatty acids and prostaglandins in alcoholic, habitually violent, and impulsive offenders', *Biological Psychiatry*, September 1987;22(9):1087–96; also C. Iribarren, et al., 'Dietary intake of n-3, n-6 fatty acids and fish: Relationship with hostility in young adults – the CARDIA study', *European Journal of Clinical Nutrition*, January 2004;58(1):24–31; also L. Buydens-Branchey, et al., 'Polyunsaturated fatty acid status and relapse vulnerability in cocaine addicts', *Psychiatry Research*, 30 August 2003;120(1):29–35; and L. Buydens-Branchey, et al., 'Polyunsaturated fatty acid status and aggression in cocaine addicts', *Drug and Alcohol Dependence*, 10 September 2003;71(3):319–23; also T. Hamazaki, et al., 'The effect of docosahexaenoic acid on aggression in elderly Thai subjects: A placebo-controlled double-blind study', *Nutritional Neuroscience*, February 2002;5(1):37–41; also M. Zanarini and F. Frankenburg, 'Omega-3 fatty acid treatment of women with borderline personality disorder: A double-blind, placebo-controlled pilot study', *American Journal of Psychiatry*, January 2003;160(1):167–9; also T. Hamazaki and S. Hirayama, 'The effect of docosahexaenoic acid-containing food administration on symptoms of attention-deficit/hyperactivity disorder: A placebo-controlled double-blind study', *European Journal of Clinical Nutrition*, 2004 May;58(5):8388; also M. Itomura, et al., 'The effect of fish oil on physical aggression in schoolchildren: A randomized, double-blind, placebo-controlled trial', *Journal of Nutritional Biochemistry*, March 2005;16(3):163–71

42 N. V. Kraguljac, et al., 'Efficacy of omega-3 Fatty acids in mood disorders: A systematic review and metaanalysis', *Psychopharmacology Bulletin*, 2009;42(3):39–54; also P. Lin and K. Su, 'A meta-analytic review of double-blind, placebo-controlled trials of antidepressant efficacy of omega-3 fatty acids', *Journal of Clinical Psychiatry*, 2007 Jul;68(7):1056–61

43 I. Cernak, et al., 'Alterations in magnesium and oxidative status during chronic emotional stress', *Magnesium Research*, 2000;13:29–36

44 P. G. Weston, 'Magnesium as a sedative', *American Journal of Psychiatric Rehabilitation*, 1921;78:637–8

45 G. A. Eby, et al., 'Rapid recovery from major depression using magnesium treatment', *Medical Hypotheses*, 2006; 67(2):362–70

46 M. Nechifor, 'Magnesium in major depression', *Magnesium Research*, 2009 September;22(3):163S–6S

47 B. Szewczyk, et al., 'Antidepressant activity of zinc and magnesium in view of the current hypotheses of antidepressant action', *Pharmacological Reports*, September–October 2008;60(5):588–9

48 B. Szewczyk, et al., 'The involvement of serotonergic system in the antidepressant effect of zinc in the forced swim test', *Progress in Neuro-psychopharmacology and Biological Psychiatry*, 17 March 2009;33(2):323–9

49 M. Siwek, et al., 'Zinc supplementation augments efficacy of imipramine in treatment resistant patients: A double blind, placebo-controlled study', *Journal of Affective Disorders*, November 2009;118(1–3):187–95, Department of Psychiatry, Collegium Medicum, Jagiellonian University, Kraków, Poland

50 W. McGinnis, et al., 'Discerning the mauve factor, Part 1', *Alternative Therapies in Health and Medicine*, March–April 2008;14(2):40–50; also see W. R. McGinnis, et al., 'Discerning the mauve factor, Part 2', *Alternative Therapies in Health and Medicine*, May–June 2008;14(3):56–62

51 J. Docherty, et al., 'A double-blind, placebo-controlled, exploratory trial of chromium picolinate in atypical depression', *Journal of Psychiatric Practice*, 2005;11(5):302–14

52 J. R. Davidson, et al., 'Effectiveness of chromium in atypical depression: A placebo-controlled trial', *Biological Psychiatry*, 1 February 2003;53(3):261–4

53 Personal communication, by email

54 K. Linde, et al., 'St John's wort for major depression', *Cochrane Database of Systematic Reviews*, 2008 Oct 8;(4):CD000448

Part 2

55 G. Reaven, 'Role of insulin resistance in human disease', *Diabetes*, 1988;37:1595–1607

56 G. P. Chrousos and T. Kino, 'Glucocorticoid signalling in the cell: Expanding clinical implications to complex human behavioural and somatic disorders', *Annals of the New York Academy of Sciences*, October 2009;1179:153–66

57 R. S. McIntyre, et al., 'Should depressive syndromes be reclassified as "Metabolic Syndrome Type II"?', *Annals of Clinical Psychiatry*, October–December 2007;19(4):257:64

58 H. Koponen, et al., 'Metabolic syndrome predisposes to depressive symptoms: A population-based 7-year follow-up study', *Journal of Clinical Psychiatry*, February 2008;69(2):178–82

59 L. Pulkki-Raback, et al., 'Depressive symptoms and the metabolic syndrome in childhood and adulthood: A prospective cohort study', *Health Psychology*, 28 January 2009;(1):108–16

60 O. P. Almeida, et al., 'Obesity and metabolic syndrome increase the risk of incident depression in older men: The health in men study', *American Journal of Geriatric Psychiatry*, October 2009;17(10):889–98

61 T. Takeuchi, et al., 'Association of metabolic syndrome with depression and anxiety in Japanese men: A one year cohort study', *Diabetic Medicine*, February 2009;35(1):32–6

62   E. M. Goldbacher, et al., 'Lifetime history of major depression predicts the development of the metabolic syndrome in middle-aged women', *Psychosomatic Medicine*, April 2009;71(3):266–72

63   M. Vanhala, et al., 'Depressive symptoms predispose females to metabolic syndrome: A 7-year follow-up study', *Acta Psychiatrica Scandinavica*, February 2009;119(2):137–42; also, H. Viinamaki, et al., 'Association of depressive symptoms and metabolic syndrome in men', *Acta Psychiatrica Scandinavica*, July 2009;120(1):23–9

64   A. Pan, et al., 'Insulin resistance and depressive symptoms in middle-aged and elderly Chinese: Findings from the Nutrition and Health of Aging Population in China Study', *Journal of Affective Disorders*, July 2008;109(1–2):75–82

65   L. K. Richardson, et al., 'Longitudinal effects of depression on glycemic control in veterans with Type 2 diabetes', *General Hospital Psychiatry*, November–December 2008;30(6):509–14. Epub 11 September 2008

66   C. R. Gale, et al, 'Fasting glucose, diagnosis of type 2 diabetes, and depression: the Vietnam experience study', *Biological Psychiatry*, 2010 January 15;67(2):189–92

67   R. Wurtman and J. Wurtman, 'Carbohydrates and depression', *Scientific American*, January 1989;260(1):68–75

68   D. E. Thomas, et al., 'Low glycemic index or low glycemic load diets for overweight and obesity', *Cochrane Database of Systematic Reviews*, 18 July 2007;(3):CD005105. Review

69   G. D. Brinkworth, et al., 'Long-term effects of a very low-carbohydrate diet and a low-fat diet on mood and cognitive function', *Archives of Internal Medicine*, 9 November 2009;169(20):1873–80

70   A. R. Cheatham, et al., 'Long-term effects of provided low and high glycemic load low energy diets on mood and cognition', *Physiology and Behaviour,* 2009 September 7;98(3):374–9

71   P. Holford, et al., '100% Health Survey', Holford & Associates Ltd

72   M. McLeod, et al., 'Effectiveness of chromium in atypical depression: A placebo-controlled trial', *Biological Psychiatry*, 2003; 53(3):261–4

73   A. Piotrowska, et al., 'Antidepressant-like effect of chromium chloride in the mouse forced swim test: Involvement of glutamatergic and serotonergic receptors', *Pharmacological Reports,* November–December 2008;60(6):991–5

74   M. McLeod, et al., 'Chromium potentiation of antidepressant pharmacotherapy for dysthymic disorder in 5 patients', *Journal of Clinical Psychiatry*, April 1999;60(4):237

75   A. Nierenberg, et al., 'Clinical and demographic features of atypical depression in outpatients with major depressive disorder: Preliminary findings from STAR*D', *Journal of Clinical Psychiatry*, 2005;66(8):1002–11

76   J. Davidson, et al., 'Effectiveness of chromium in atypical depression: A placebo-controlled trial', *Biological Psychiatry*, 2003;53(3):261–4

77   J. Docherty, et al., 'A double-blind, placebo-controlled, exploratory trial of

chromium picolinate in atypical depression', *Journal of Psychiatric Practice*, 2005;11(5):302–14

78   A. Jabbar, et al., 'Vitamin B$_{12}$ deficiency common in primary hypothyroidism', *Journal of the Pakistan Medical Association*, May 2008;58(5):258–61

79   J. C. Toft and H. Toft, 'Hyperhomocysteinemia and hypothyroidism', *Ugeskrift for Laeger* (Denmark), 2001;163(34):4593–4

80   W. I. Hussein, et al., 'Normalization of hyperhomocysteinemia with L-thyroxine in hypothyroidism', *Annals of Internal Medicine*, 7 September 1999;131(5):348–51; also M. Bicikova, et al., 'Effect of treatment of hypothyroidism on the plasma concentrations of neuroactive steroids and homocysteine', *Clinical Chemistry and Laboratory Medicine*, 2001;39(8):753–7

81   A. Jabbar, et al., 'Vitamin B$_{12}$ deficiency common in primary hypothyroidism', *Journal of the Pakistan Medical Association*, May 2008;58(5):258–61

82   G. A. Colditz, et al., 'The use of estrogens and progestins and the risk of breast cancer in postmenopausal women', *New England Journal of Medicine*, 1995;332(24):1589–93

83   E. Barrett-Connor, et al., 'Bioavailable testosterone and depressed mood in older men: The Rancho Bernardo Study', *Journal of Clinical Endocrinology and Metabolism*, 1999;84(2):573–794

84   O. M. Wolkowitz, et al., 'Dehydroepiandrosterone (DHEA) treatment of depression', *Biological Psychiatry*, 1997;41(3):311–18

85   A. N. Margioris, 'Fatty acids and postprandial inflammation', *Current Opinion in Clinical Nutrition & Metabolic Care*, 2009;12(2):129–37

86   D. Benton, et al., 'Impact of consuming a milk drink containing a probiotic on mood and cognition', *European Journal of Clinical Nutrition*, 2007;61(3):355–61

87   F. Barreau, et al., 'Neonatal maternal deprivation triggers long term alterations in colonic epithelial barrier and mucosal immunity in rats', *Gut*, April 2004;53(4):501–6

88   M. G. Gareau, et al., 'Probiotic treatment of rat pups normalises corticosterone release and ameliorates colonic dysfunction induced by maternal separation', *Gut*, 2007;56:1522–8

89   G. Meloni, et al., 'Subclinical coeliac disease in schoolchildren from northern Sardinia', *Lancet*, 2 January 1999;353(9146):37

90   C. Ciacci, et al., 'Depressive symptoms in adult coeliac disease', *Scandinavian Journal of Gastroenterology*, March 1998;33(3):247–50

91   R. P. Ford, 'The gluten syndrome: A neurological disease', *Medical Hypotheses*, September 2009;73(3):438–40

92   T. Randolph, 'Allergy as a causative factor of fatigue, irritability and behaviour problems of children', *Journal of Paediatrics*, 1947;31:560; A. Rowe, 'Allergic toxemia and fatigue', *Annals of Allergy*, 1959;17:9; G. Speer, *Allergy of the Nervous System*, 1970, Thomas; M. Campbell, 'Neurologic manifestations of allergic disease', *Annals of Allergy*, 1973;31:485; K. Hall, 'Allergy of the nervous

system: A review', *Annals of Allergy*, 1976;36:49–64; V. Pippere, 'Some varieties of food intolerance in psychiatric patients', *Nutrition and Health*, 1984;3:125–36; C. Pfeiffer and P. Holford, *Mental Illness and Schizophrenia: The Nutrition Connection*, 1989, Thorsons; T. Tuormaa, *An Alternative to Psychiatry*, 1991, The Book Guild; G. Parker and T. Watkins, 'Treatment-resistant depression: When antidepressant drug intolerance may indicate food intolerance', *Australian and New Zealand Journal of Psychiatry*, April 2002;36(2):263–5

93   J. Egger, et al., 'Controlled trial of oligoantigenic diet treatment in the hyperkinetic syndrome', *Lancet*, 1985;1:540–5

94   B. Feingold, 'Dietary management of behaviour and learning disabilities', *Nutrition and Behaviour*, S. A. Miller (ed), 1981, Franklin Institute Press

95   C. Roos, et al., 'A discriminating messenger RNA signature for bipolar disorder formed by an aberrant expression of inflammatory genes in monocytes', *Archives of General Psychiatry*, 2008;65(4):395–407; also see S. Zeugmann, et al., 'Inflammatory biomarkers in 70 depressed inpatients with and without the metabolic syndrome', *Journal of Clinical Psychiatry*, 9 February 2010; also see B. Fang, et al., 'Disturbed sleep: Linking allergic rhinitis, mood and suicidal behavior', *Frontiers of Bioscience*, 1 January 2010;2:30–46

96   K. Lillestøl, et al., 'Anxiety and depression in patients with self-reported food hypersensitivity', *General Hospital Psychiatry*, January–February 2010;32(1):42–8

97   S. Zar, et al., 'Food-specific serium IgG4 and IgE titers to common food antigens in irritable bowel syndrome', *American Journal of Gastroenterology*, 2005;100:1550–7

98   W. Atkinson, et al., 'Food elimination based on IgG antibodies in irritable bowel syndrome: A randomized controlled trial', *Gut*, October 2004;53(10):1459–64

99   G. Hardman and G. Hart, 'Dietary advice based on food specific IgG results', *Nutrition and Food Science*, 2007; 37:16–23 plus further analysis of data provided by the author

100   J. R. Hibbeln, 'Seafood consumption and homicide mortality: A cross-national ecological analysis', *World Review of Nutrition and Dietetics*, 2001;88:41–6

101   J. R. Hibbeln, 'Fish consumption and major depression', *Lancet*, 1998;351:1213; also J. R. Hibbeln, 'Depression, suicide and deficiencies of omega-3 essential fatty acids in modern diets', *World Review of Nutrition and Dietetics*, 2009;99:17–30; see also J. R. Hibbeln, 'From homicide to happiness: A commentary on omega-3 fatty acids in human society. Cleave Award Lecture', *Nutrition and Health*, 2007;19(1–2):9–19

102   B. Hallahan, et al., 'Omega-3 fatty acid supplementation in patients with recurrent self-harm: Single-centre double-blind randomised controlled trial', *British Journal of Psychiatry*, February 2007;190:118–22

103   J. R. Hibbeln, et al., 'Increasing homicide rates and linoleic acid consumption among five Western countries, 1961–2000', *Lipids*, December 2004;39(12):1207–13

104   J. Golding, et al., 'High levels of depressive symptoms in pregnancy with low omega-3 fatty acid intake from fish', *Epidemiology*, July 2009;20(4):598–603

105 M. E. Virkkunen, et al., 'Plasma phospholipid essential fatty acids and prostaglandins in alcoholic, habitually violent, and impulsive offenders', *Biological Psychiatry*, September 1987;22(9):1087–96; see also C. Iribarren, et al., 'Dietary intake of n-3, n-6 fatty acids and fish: Relationship with hostility in young adults. The CARDIA study', *European Journal of Clinical Nutrition*, January 2004;58(1):24–31; see also L. Buydens-Branchey, et al., 'Polyunsaturated fatty acid status and relapse vulnerability in cocaine addicts', *Psychiatry Research*, 2003 August 30;120(1):29–35; see also L. Buydens-Branchey, et al., 'Polyunsaturated fatty acid status and aggression in cocaine addicts', *Drug and Alcohol Dependence*, 2003 Sep 10;71(3):319–23; see also T. Hamazaki, et al., 'The effect of docosahexaenoic acid on aggression in elderly Thai subjects: A placebo-controlled double-blind study', *Nutritional Neuroscience*, February 2002;5(1):37–41; M. Zanarini and F. Frankenburg, 'Omega-3 fatty acid treatment of women with borderline personality disorder: A double-blind, placebo-controlled pilot study', *American Journal of Psychiatry*, 2003 January;160(1):167–9; T. Hamazaki and S. Hirayama, 'The effect of docosahexaenoic acid-containing food administration on symptoms of attention-deficit/hyperactivity disorder: A placebo-controlled double-blind study', *European Journal of Clinical Nutrition*, May 2004;58(5):8388; M. Itomura, et al., 'The effect of fish oil on physical aggression in schoolchildren: A randomized, double-blind, placebo-controlled trial', *Journal of Nutritional Biochemistry*, March 2005;16(3):163–71

106 J. R. Hibbeln, 'Fish consumption and major depression', *Lancet*, 1998;351:1213

107 M. B. Raeder, et al., 'Associations between cod liver oil use and symptoms of depression: The Hordaland Health Study', *Journal of Affective Disorders*, August 2007;101(1–3):245:9. Epub 19 December 2006

108 P. Lin and K. Su, 'A meta-analytic review of double-blind, placebo-controlled trials of antidepressant efficacy of omega-3 fatty acids', *Journal of Clinical Psychiatry*, July 2007;68(7):1056–61; also N. V. Kraguljac, et al., 'Efficacy of omega-3 fatty acids in mood disorders: A systematic review and metaanalysis', *Psychopharmacology Bulletin*, 2009;42(3):39–54; M. Peet and C. Stokes, 'Omega-3 fatty acids in the treatment of psychiatric disorders', *Drugs*, 2005;65(8):1051–9

109 A. Stoll, 'Omega 3 fatty acids in bipolar disorder', *Archives of General Psychiatry*, 1999;56:407–12; see also B. Nemets, et al., 'Addition of omega-3 fatty acid to maintenance medication treatment for recurrent unipolar depressive disorder', *American Journal of Psychiatry*, 2002;159:477–9; Y. Osher, et al., 'Omega-3 eicosapentaenoic acid in bipolar depression: Report of a small open-label study', *Journal of Clinical Psychiatry*, June 2005;66(6):726–9

110 B. Nemets, et al., 'Addition of omega-3 fatty acid to maintenance medication treatment for recurrent unipolar depressive disorder', *American Journal of Psychiatry*, 2002;159:477–9

111 S. Frangou, et al., 'Efficacy of ethyl-eicosapentaenoic acid in bipolar depression: Randomised double-blind placebo-controlled study', *British Journal of Psychiatry*, 2006;188:46–50

112 K. P. Su, et al., 'Omega-3 fatty acids for major depressive disorder during pregnancy: Results from a randomized, double-blind, placebo-controlled trial', *Journal of Clinical Psychiatry*, April 2008;69(4):644–51

113 M. Lucas, et al., 'Ethyl-eicosapentaenoic acid for the treatment of psychological distress and depressive symptoms in middle-aged women: A double-blind, placebo-controlled, randomized clinical trial', *American Journal of Clinical Nutrition*, February 2009;89(2):641–51

114 E. C. Suarez, 'Relations of trait depression and anxiety to low lipid and lipoprotein concentrations in healthy young adult women', *Psychosomatic Medicine*, 1999;61(3):273–9

115 T. Partonen, et al., 'Association of low serum total cholesterol with major depression and suicide', *British Journal of Psychiatry*, 1999;175:259–62

116 A. Margioris, 'Fatty acids and postprandial inflammation', *Current Opinion in Clinical Nutrition and Metabolic Care*, March 2009;12(2):129–37; also P. Lin and K. Su, 'A meta-analytic review of double-blind, placebo-controlled trials of antidepressant efficacy of omega-3 fatty acids', *Journal of Clinical Psychiatry*, July 2007;68(7):1056–61

117 R. J. Goldberg and J. Katz, 'A meta-analysis of the analgesic effects of omega-3 polyunsaturated fatty acid supplementation for inflammatory joint pain', *Pain*, May 2007;129(1–2):210–23

118 No authors listed, 'Dietary supplementation with n-3 polyunsaturated fatty acids and vitamin E after myocardial infarction: Results of the GISSI-Prevenzione trial', *Lancet*, 7 August 1999;354(9177):447–55; also P. M. Kris-Etherton, et al., 'Fish consumption, fish oil, omega-3 fatty acids and cardiovascular disease', *Circulation*, 19 November 2002;106(21):2747–57; American Heart Association Nutrition Committee, et al., 'Diet and lifestyle recommendations revision 2006: A scientific statement from the American Heart Association Nutrition Committee', *Circulation*, 4 July 2006;114(1):82–96

119 No authors listed, 'Dietary supplementation with n-3 polyunsaturated fatty acids and vitamin E after myocardial infarction: Results of the GISSI-Prevenzione trial', *Lancet*, 7 August 1999;354(9177):447–55

120 J. A. Simon, et al., 'Serum fatty acids and the risk of coronary heart disease', *American Journal of Epidemiology*, 1 September 1995;142(5):469–76

121 V. Bountziouka, et al., 'Long-term fish intake is associated with less severe depressive symptoms among elderly men and women: The MEDIS (MEDiterranean ISlands Elderly) epidemiological study', *Journal of Aging and Health*, September 2009;21(6):864–80

122 L. A. Colangelo, et al., 'Higher dietary intake of long-chain omega-3 polyunsaturated fatty acids is inversely associated with depressive symptoms in women', *Nutrition*, October 2009;25(10):1011–19

123 J. Golding, et al., 'High levels of depressive symptoms in pregnancy with low omega-3 fatty acid intake from fish', *Epidemiology*, July 2009; 20(4):598–603

124 A. Dubini, et al., 'Do noradrenaline & serotonin differentially affect social motivation and behaviour?', *European Neuropsychopharmacology*, 1997; 7(Suppl): S49–S55

125 G. R. Heninger, 'Serotonin, sex, psychiatric illness', *Proceedings of the National Academy of Sciences of the United States of America*, 1997;94(4):823–4

126 J. Shepherd, 'Effects of estrogen on cognition, mood and degenerative brain diseases', *Journal of the American Pharmaceutical Association (Washington D. C.)*, 2001;41(2):221–8

127 K. A. Smith, et al., 'Relapse of depression after rapid depletion of tryptophan', *Lancet*, 1997;349:915–19

128 I. von Sano, 'L-5-Hydroxytryptophan (L-5-HTP) therapie', *Folia Psychiatrica et Neurologica Japonica*, 1972;26(1):7–17; see also T. Nakajima, et al., 'Clinical evaluation of 5-hydroxy-L-tryptophan as an antidepressant drug', *Folia Psychiatrica et Neurologica Japonica*, 1978;32(2):225ff; E. H. Turner, et al. 'Serotonin a la carte: Supplementation with the serotonin precursor 5-hydroxytryptophan', *Pharmacology and Therapeutics*, 2006;109(3):325–38; W. Poldinger, et al., 'A functional-dimensional approach to depression: Serotonin deficiency and target syndrome in a comparison of 5-hydroxytryptophan and fluvoxamine', *Psychopathology*, 1991;24(2):53–81; A. Woggon and J. Schoef, 'The treatment of depression with L-5-Hydroxytryptophan versus Imipramine', *Archiv fur Psychiatrie und Nervenkrankheiten*, 1977;224:175–86; T. Nakajima, et al., 'Clinical evaluation of 5-hydroxy-L-tryptophan as an antidepressant drug', *Folia Psychiatrica et Neurologica Japonica*, 1978;32(2):223–30; M. van Praag, et al., 'A pilot study of the predictive value of the probnecid test in application of 5-hydroxytryptophan as antidepressant', *Psychopharmacologica (Berlin)*, 1972;25:14–21; M. Kaneko, et al., 'L-5-HTP treatment and serum 5-HT level after L-5-HTP loading on depressed patients', *Neuropsychobiology*, 1979;5:232–40; see also L. J. van Heile, 'L-5-hydroxytryptophan in depression: The first substitution therapy in psychiatry?', *Neuropsychobiology*, 1980;6:230–40

129 T. Nakajima, et al., 'Clinical evaluation of 5-hydroxy-L-tryptophan as an antidepressant drug', *Folia Psychiatrica et Neurologica*, 1978;32(2):225ff

130 W. Poldinger, et al., 'A functional-dimensional approach to depression: Serotonin deficiency and target syndrome in a comparison of 5-hydroxytryptophan and fluvoxamine', *Psychopathology*, 1991;24(2):53–81

131 A. Woggon and J. Schoef, 'The treatment of depression with L-5-hydroxytryptophan versus imipramine', *Archiv fur Psychiatrie und Nervenkrankheiten*, 1977;224:175–86

132 T. Nakajima, et al., 'Clinical evaluation of 5-hydroxy-L-tryptophan as an antidepressant drug', *Folia Psychiatrica et Neurologica Japonica*, 1978;32(2):223–230; M. van Praag, et al., 'A pilot study of the predictive value of the probnecid test in application of 5-Hydroxytryptophan as antidepressant', *Psychopharmacologica (Berlin)*, 1972;25:14–21; M. Kaneko, et al., 'L-5-HTP treatment and serum 5-HT level after L-5-HTP loading on depressed patients', *Neuropsychobiology*,

1979;5:232–40; L. J. van Heile, 'L-5-hydroxytryptophan in depression: The first substitution therapy in psychiatry?', *Neuropsychobiology*, 1980;6:230–40; and I. von Sano, 'L-5-hydroxytryptophan (L-5-HTP) therapie', *Folia Psychiatrica et Neurologica Japonica*, 1972;26(1):7–17

133 T. C. Birdsall, '5-Hydroxytryptophan: A clinically-effective serotonin precursor', *Alternative Medicine Review*, August 1998;3(4):271–80

134 E. H. Turner, et al., 'Serotonin a la carte: Supplementation with the serotonin precursor 5-hydroxytryptophan', *Pharmacology & Therapeutics*, 2006;109(3):325–38

135 Y. T. Das, et al., 'Safety of 5-hydroxy-L-tryptophan', *Toxicology Letter*, 15 April 2004;150(1):111–22

136 T. Audhya, 'Advances in measurement of platelet catecholamines at sub-picomole level for diagnosis of depression and anxiety', *Clinical Chemistry*, 2005;51(6) supplement, E-128

137 ibid.

138 Conference presentation at Annual Meeting of American Association of Clinical Chemistry, 2005

139 H. Beckmann, et al., 'DL-phenylalanine versus imipramine: A double-blind controlled study', *Archiv fur Psychiatrie und Nervenkrankheiten*, 1979; 227(1):49–58

140 H. C. Sabelli, et al., 'Clinical studies on the phenylethylamine hypothesis of affective disorder: Urine and blood phenylacetic acid and phenylalanine dietary supplements', *The Journal of Clinical Psychiatry*, 1986;(2):66–70

141 J. Mouret, et al., 'L-tyrosine cures, immediate and long term, dopamine-dependent depressions: Clinical and polygraphic studies', *Comptes rendus de l'Academie des sciences. Serie III, Sciences de la vie*, 1988;306(3):93–8 (in French)

142 J. B. Deijen, et al., 'Tyrosine improves cognitive performance and reduces blood pressure in cadets after one week of a combat training course', *Brain Research Bulletin*, 1999; 48(2):203–9

143 C. R. Mahoney, et al., 'Tyrosine supplementation mitigates working memory decrements during cold exposure', *Physiology and Behaviour*, 23 November 2007;92(4):575–82

144 S. F. McTavish, et al., 'Lack of effect of tyrosine depletion on mood in recovered depressed women', *Neuropsychopharm*, 2005;30(4):786–91

145 T. Audhya, 'Advances in measurement of platelet catecholamines at sub-picomole level for diagnosis of depression and anxiety', *Clinical Chemistry*, 2005;51(6) supplement, E-128

146 D. J. Easty and D. C. Bennett, 'Protein tyrosine kinases in malignant melanoma', *Melanoma Research*, October 2000;10(5):401–11

147 M. J. Sole, et al., 'Chronic dietary tyrosine supplements do not affect mild essential hypertension', *Hypertension*, 1985 July–Aug;7(4):593–6

148 K. M. Bell, et al., 'S-adenosylmethionine treatment of depression: A clinical trial', *American Journal of Psychiatry*, 1988;145:110–14

149 M. Fava, et al., 'Rapidity of onset of the antidepressant effect of parenteral S-adenosyl-L-methionine', *Psychiatry Research*, 28 April 1995;56(3):295–7; also P. G. Janicak, et al., 'Parenteral S-adenosylmethionine in depression: A literature review and preliminary report', *Psychopharmacology Bulletin*, 1989;25:238–41

150 M. De Vanna and R. Rigamonti, 'Oral S-adenosyl-L-methionine in depression', *Current Therapeutic Research, Clinical And Experimental*, 1992;52:478–85

151 P. Salmaggi, et al., 'Double-blind, placebo-controlled study of S-adenosyl-L-methionine in depressed postmenopausal women', *Psychotherapy and Psychosomatics*, 1993;59:34–40

152 F. L. Kagan, et al., 'Oral S-adenosylmethionine in depression: A randomized, double-blind placebo-controlled trial', *American Journal of Psychiatry*, 1990;147:591–5

153 G. M. Bressa, 'S-adenosyl-methionine as antidepressant: Meta-analysis of clinical studies', *Acta Neurologica Scandinavica*, 1994;154(supp):7–14

154 I. Caruso and V. Pietrogrande, 'Italian double-blind multicenter study comparing S-adenosylmethionine, naproxen and placebo in the treatment of degenerative joint disease', *American Journal of Medicine*, 1987 November 20;83(5A):66–71

155 S. H. Zeisel, et al., 'Concentrations of choline-containing compounds and betaine in common foods', *Journal of Nutrition*, May 2003;133(5):1302–7. Erratum in: *Journal of Nutrition*, 2003 Sep;133(9):2918

156 Q. Regestein, et al., 'Sleep debt and depression in female college students', *Psychiatry Research*, 30 March 2010;176(1):34–9

157 A. Brzezinski, et al., 'Effects of exogenous melatonin on sleep: A meta-analysis', *Sleep Medicine Reviews*, 2005;9(1):41–50

158 S. A. Rahman, et al., 'Antidepressant action of melatonin in the treatment of Delayed Sleep Phase Syndrome', *Sleep Medicine*, February 2010;11(2):131–6

159 T. C. Birdsall, '5-Hydroxytryptophan: A clinically-effective serotonin precursor', *Alternative Medicine Review*, 1998;3(4):271–80

160 O. Bruni, et al., 'L-5-Hydroxytryptophan treatment of sleep terrors in children', *European Journal of Pediatric Neurology*, 2004;163(7):402–7

161 S. Young, 'The Clinical Psychopharmacology of Tryptophan', in J. and R. Wurtman (eds), *Nutrition and the Brain*, 1986, Raven Press, New York

162 C. Baglioni, et al., 'Sleep and emotions: A focus on insomnia', *Sleep Medicine Reviews*, 3 February 2010 (Epub ahead of print)

163 L. Shilo, et al., 'The effects of coffee consumption on sleep and melatonin secretion', *Sleep Medicine*, 2002;3(3):271–3

164 W. Shell, et al., 'A randomized, placebo-controlled trial of an amino acid preparation on timing and quality of sleep', *American Journal of Therapeutics*, 15 May 2009

165 M. Hornyak, 'Magnesium therapy for periodic leg movements-related insomnia and restless legs syndrome: An open pilot study', *Sleep*, 1998;21(5):501–5

166 M. Spinella, *The Psychopharmacology of Herbal Medicine*, 2001, MIT Press, London

167 M. Dorn, 'Valerian versus oxazepam: Efficacy and tolerability in nonorganic and nonpsychiatric insomniacs – a randomized, double-blind clinical comparative study', *Forschende Komplementarmedizin und Klassiche naturheilkunde*, 2000;7:79–81

168 E. Vorbach, et al., 'Treatment of Insomnia: Effectiveness and tolerance of a valerian extract', *Psychopharmakotheraphie*,1996;3:109–15

169 S. Bent, et al., 'Valerian for sleep: A systematic review and meta-analysis', *American Journal of Medicine*, December 2006;119(12):1005–12. Review

170 L. Yai, '"Brain music" in the treatment of patients with insomnia', *Neuroscience and Behavioural Physiology*, 1998;28:330–5

171 I. Olszewska and M. Zarow, 'Does music during dental treatment make a difference?' See: www.silenceofmusic.com/pdf/dentists.pdf

172 G. D. Jacobs, et al., 'Cognitive behaviour therapy and pharmacotherapy for insomnia: A randomized controlled trial and direct comparison', *Archives of Internal Medicine*, 2004;164(17):1888–96

173 H. Tiemeier, et al., 'Vitamin B_{12}, folate, and homocysteine in depression: the Rotterdam Study', *American Journal of Psychiatry*, 2002;159(12):2099–101; see also T. Bottiglieri, et al., 'Homocysteine, folate, methylation, and monoamine metabolism in depression', *Journal of Neurology, Neurosurgery and Psychiatry*, 2000;69:228–32; M. Fava and T. Bottiglieri, et al., 'Folate, vitamin B_{12}, and homocysteine in major depressive disorder'. *American Journal of Psychiatry*, 1997;154:426–8

174 H. Refsum, et al., 'Folate, vitamin B_{12}, homocysteine, and the MTHFR polymorphism in anxiety and depression: The Hordaland Homocysteine Study', *Archives of General Psychiatry*, 2003;60:618–26

175 T. Bottiglieri, et al., 'Homocysteine, folate, methylation, and monoamine metabolism in depression', *Journal of Neurology, Neurosurgery and Psychiatry*, 2000;69(2):228–32

176 A. Nanri, et al., 'Serum folate and homocysteine and depressive symptoms among Japanese men and women', *European Journal of Clinical Nutrition*, March 2010;64(3):289–96

177 S. Gilbody, et al., 'Is low folate a risk factor for depression? A meta-analysis and exploration of heterogeneity', *Journal of Epidemiology and Community Health*, July 2007;61(7):631–7

178 J. M. Kim, et al., 'Predictive value of folate, vitamin B_{12} and homocysteine levels in late life depression', *British Journal of Psychiatry*, April 2008;192(4):268–74; also see N. Dimopoulos, et al., 'Correlation of folate, vitamin B_{12} and homocysteine plasma levels with depression in an elderly Greek population', *Clinical Biochemistry*, June 2007;40(9–10):604–8; see also P. S. Sachdev, et al., 'Relationship of homocysteine, folic acid and vitamin B_{12} with depression in a middle-aged community sample', *Psychological Medicine*, April 2005;35(4):529–38; A. Coppen and C. Bolander-Gouaille, 'Treatment of depression: Time to consider folic acid and vitamin B_{12}', *Journal of Psychopharmacology*, January 2005;19(1):59–65. Review

179 A. M. Hvas, et al., 'Vitamin B$_6$ level is associated with symptoms of depression', *Psychotherapy and Psychosomatics*, November–December 2004;73(6):340–3

180 A. Coppen and C. Bolander-Gouaille, 'Treatment of depression: Time to consider folic acid and vitamin B$_{12}$', *Journal of Psychopharmacology*, January 2005;19(1):59–65. Review; also see J. Hintikka, et al., 'High vitamin B$_{12}$ level and good treatment outcome may be associated in major depressive disorder', *BMC Psychiatry*, 2 December 2003;3:17

181 S. Gariballa and S. Forster, 'Effects of dietary supplements on depressive symptoms in older patients: A randomised double-blind placebo-controlled trial', *Clinical Nutrition*, October 2007;26(5):545–51

182 M. Morris et al., 'Depression and folate status in the US population', *Psychotherapy and Psychosomatics*, 2003;72:80–7; see also M. J. Taylor, et al., 'Folate for depressive disorders', *Cochrane Database of Systematic Reviews*, 2003;2: Art. No: CD003390. DOI: 10.1002/14651858.CD003390.

183 A. Coppen and J. Bailey, 'Enhancement of the antidepressant action of fluoxetine by folic acid: A randomised, placebo controlled trial', *Affective Disorders*, 2000;60:121–30

184 A. Vogiatzoglou, et al., 'Vitamin B$_{12}$ status and rate of brain volume loss in community-dwelling elderly', *Neurology*, 2008;71:826–32

185 T. P. Ng, et al., ' Folate, vitamin B$_{12}$, homocysteine, and depressive symptoms in a population sample of older Chinese adults', *Journal of the American Geriatrics Society*, May 2009;57(5):871–6

186 N. J. Marini, et al., 'The prevalence of folate-remedial MTHFR enzyme variants in humans', *Proceedings of the National Academy of Sciences*, 10 June 2008;105(23):8055–60

187 A. Vogiatzoglou, et al., 'Vitamin B$_{12}$ status and rate of brain volume loss in community-dwelling elderly', *Neurology*, 2008;71:826–32; see also S. J. Eussen, et al., 'Oral cyanocobalamin supplementation in older people with vitamin B$_{12}$ deficiency', *Archives of Internal Medicine*, 2005;165:1167–72

188 H. Refsum, et al., 'The Hordaland Homocysteine Study: A community-based study of homocysteine, its determinants, and associations with disease', *Journal of Nutrition*, 2006;136:1731S–1740S

189 G. W. Lambert, et al., 'Effect of sunlight and season on serotonin turnover in the brain', *Lancet*, 2002;360(9348):1840–2

190 S. Grimaldi, et al., 'Experienced poor lighting contributes to the seasonal fluctuations in weight and appetite that relate to the metabolic syndrome', *Journal of Environmental and Public Health*, 2009 June 7:165013

191 R. N. Golden, et al.,'The efficacy of light therapy in the treatment of mood disorders: A review and meta-analysis of the evidence', *American Journal of Psychiatry*, 2005;162:656–62

192 K. Martiny, et al., 'Adjunctive bright light in non-seasonal major depression: Results from clinician-rated depression scales', *Acta Psychiatrica Scandinavica*, 2005;112(2):117–25

193 L. Swiecicki, et al., 'Platelet serotonin transport in the group of outpatients with seasonal affective disorder before and after light treatment, and in remission (in the summer)', *Psychiatria Polska*, 2005;39(3):459–68

194 C. Wilkins, et al., 'Vitamin D deficiency is associated with low mood and worse cognitive performance in older adults', *The American Journal of Geriatric Psychiatry*, 2006;14(12):1032–40; see also W. J. Hoogendijk, et al., 'Depression is associated with decreased 25-hydroxyvitamin D and increased parathyroid hormone levels in older adults', *Journal of Internal Medicine*, 2008 December;264(6):599–609; see also A. Nanri, et al., 'Association between serum 25-hydroxyvitamin D and depressive symptoms in Japanese: analysis by survey season', *European Journal of Clinical Nutrition*, 2009 December;63(12):1444–7: see also D. J. Armstrong, et al., 'Vitamin D deficiency is associated with anxiety and depression in fibromyalgia', *Clinical Rheumatology*, 2007;26:551–4; see also A. T. Lansdowne and S. C. Provost, 'Vitamin D₃ enhances mood in healthy subjects during winter', *Psychopharmacology (Berlin)*, 1998;135:319–23

195 R. Jorde, et al., 'Effects of vitamin D supplementation on symptoms of depression in overweight and obese subjects: Randomized double blind trial', *Archives of General Psychiatry*, May 2008;65(5):508–12

196 A. Lansdowne and S. Provost, 'Vitamin D₃ enhances mood in healthy subjects during winter', *Psychopharmacology*, 1998;135:319–23

197 C. D. Shipowick, et al., 'Vitamin D and depressive symptoms in women during the winter: A pilot study', *Applied Nursing Research*, August 2009;22(3):221–5

198 V. Mocanu, et al., 'Long-term effects of giving nursing home residents bread fortified with 125 microg (5000 IU) vitamin D(3) per daily serving', *American Journal of Clinical Nutrition*, 2009;89(4):1132–7; see also J. F. Aloia, et al., 'Vitamin D intake to attain a desired serum 25-hydroxyvitamin D concentration', *American Journal of Clinical Nutrition*, 2008;87(6):1952–8

199 L. Craft, et al., 'The benefits of exercise for the clinically depressed', *Primary Care Companion to the Journal of Clinical Psychiatry*, 2004;6:104–11

200 N. A. Singh, 'A randomized controlled trial of high versus low intensity weight training versus general practitioner care for clinical depression in older adults', *Journals of Gerontology. Series A, Biological Sciences and Medical Sciences*, 2005;60:768–76

201 D. Kritz-Silverstein, et al., 'Cross-sectional and prospective study of exercise and depressed mood in the elderly: The Rancho Bernardo study', *American Journal of Epidemiology*, 2001;153(6):596–603

202 S. Leppamaki, et al., 'Drop-out and mood improvement: A randomised controlled trial with light exposure and physical exercise', *BMC Psychiatry*, 2004;4(1):22

203 S. Brand, et al., 'High exercise levels are related to favourable sleep patterns and psychological functioning in adolescents: A comparison of athletes and controls', *Journal of Adolescent Health*, February 2010;46(2):133–41

204 P. Montgomery and J. Dennis, 'Physical exercise for sleep problems in adults aged 60+', *Cochrane Review*, 2005; 4:The Cochrane Library

205 H. Woelk, 'Comparison of St. John's Wort and imipramine for treating depression: Randomised controlled trial', *British Medical Journal*, 2000;321, 72600:536–9

206 K. Linde, et al., 'St John's Wort for major depression', *Cochrane Database of Systematic Reviews*, 8 October 2008;(4):CD000448

207 U. Schmidt and H. Sommer, 'St. John's Wort extract in the ambulatory therapy of depression', *Fortschritte der Medizin*, 1993;111(19):339–42 (in German)

208 S. Bratman, *Beat Depression with St. John's Wort*, 1997, Prima Publishing

209 F. Borrelli and A. A. Izzo, 'Herb–drug interactions with St John's wort (Hypericum perforatum): An update on clinical observations', *AAPS Journal*, December 2009;11(4):710–27; see also J. Sarris and D. J. Kavanagh, 'Kava and St. John's wort: Current evidence for use in mood and anxiety disorders', *Journal of Alternative and Complementary Medicine*, August 2009;15(8):827–36

210 A. Brattstrom, 'Long-term effects of St. John's wort (Hypericum perforatum) treatment: A 1-year safety study in mild to moderate depression', *Phytomedicine* April 2009;16(4):277–83

211 S. Kasper, et al., 'Placebo controlled continuation treatment with Hypericum extract WS 5570 after recovery from a mild or moderate depressive episode', *Wiener medizinische Wochenschrift*, 2007;157(13–14):362–6. Department of Psychiatry and Psychotherapy, Medical University Vienna, Austria. sci-genpsy@meduniwien.ac.at

212 C. Hart, et al., 'Effect of conjugal bereavement on mortality of the bereaved spouse in participants of the Renfrew/Paisley Study', *Journal of Epidemiology and Community Health*, May 2007;61(5):455–60; see also N. Christakis and P. Allison, 'Mortality after the hospitalization of a spouse', *New England Journal of Medicine*, 16 February 2006;354(7):719–30

213 R. Churchill, et al., 'A systematic review of controlled trials of the effectiveness of brief psychological treatments for depression', *Health Technology Assessment*, 2001;5(35) (www.hta.ac.uk/execsumm/summ535.htm)

214 S. D. Hollon, et al., 'Prevention of relapse following cognitive therapy vs medications in moderate to severe depression', *Archives of General Psychiatry*, April 2005;62(4):417–22

215 A. Chiesa and A. Serretti, 'A systematic review of neurobiological and clinical features of mindfulness meditations', *Psychological Medicine*, 27 November 2009:1–14

216 J. Lagopoulos, et al., 'Increased theta and alpha EEG activity during nondirective meditation', *Journal of Alternative and Complementary Medicine*, November 2009;15(11):1187–92

217 D. Goleman, *Emotional Intelligence*, 1996 Bloomsbury

Part 3

218 L. Moisey, et al., 'Caffeinated coffee consumption impairs blood glucose homeostasisin response to high and low glycemic index meals in healthy men', *Journal of Clinical Nutrition*, 2008;87:1254–61

219 E. Cheraskin, 'The breakfast/lunch/dinner ritual', *Journal of Orthomolecular Medicine*, 1993;8:1st Quarter

220 L. A. Uebelacker, et al., 'Hatha yoga for depression: Critical review of the evidence for efficacy, plausible mechanisms of action, and directions for future research', *Journal of Psychiatric Practice*, January 2010;16(1):22–33; see also P. Posadzki, et al., 'Yoga and qigong in the psychological prevention of mental health disorders: A conceptual synthesis', *Chinese Journal of Integrative Medicine*, February 2010;16(1):80–6; M. Javnbakht, 'Effects of yoga on depression and anxiety of women', *Complementary Therapy in Clinical Practice*, May 2009;15(2):102–4

RECOMMENDED READING

General

Patrick Holford, *The Optimum Nutrition Bible*, Piatkus (2009)

Patrick Holford, *The 10 Secrets of 100% Healthy People*, Piatkus (2009)

Patrick Holford, *Optimum Nutrition for the Mind*, Piatkus (2007)

Part one – The anatomy of feeling good

Chapter 1

Paul Gilbert, *Overcoming Depression*, Robinson (2000)

Chapter 2

Gerald Jampolsky, *Love is Letting Go of Fear*, Celestial Arts (2004)

Tim Laurence, *You Can Change Your Life*, Mobius (2004)

Ksemaraja, *The Doctrine of Recognition*, State University of New York Press (1990)

Eckhart Tolle, *The Power of Now*, New World Library (2009)

Chapter 4

Irving Kirsch, *The Emperor's New Drugs*, Basic Books (2010)

Chapter 6

Patrick Holford, *The Low-GL Diet Bible*, Piatkus (2009)

Part two – My top ten mood-boosting secrets

Chapter 9

Patrick Holford and Dr James Braly, *Hidden Food Allergies,* Piatkus (2005)

Chapter 12

Joe Griffin and Ivan Tyrrell, *How to Lift Depression*, Human Givens Publishing (2007)

Chapter 15

Dr Hyla Cass, *St John's Wort: Nature's Blues Buster*, Avery Publishing (1997)

Chapter 16

Thomas Moore, *Dark Nights of the Soul*, Piatkus (2004)

Thomas Moore, *Care of the Soul*, HarperPerennial (1994)

Dennis Greenberger and Christine Padesky, *Mind Over Mood*, Guilford Press (1995)

Mark Williams et al., *The Mindful Way Through Depression*, Guilford Press (2007)

Byron Katie, *Who Would You Be Without Your Story?* Hay House (2008)

Daniel Goleman, *Emotional Intelligence*, Bantam (1997)

Patrick Holford, *The 10 Secrets of 100% Healthy People*, Piatkus (2009)

Laurel Mellin, *Wired for Joy*, Hay House (2010)

Part Three – Your mood-boosting action plan

Chapter 17

Patrick Holford and Fiona McDonald Joyce, *Food Glorious Food*, Piatkus (2008)

Patrick Holford and Judy Ridgway, *The Optimum Nutrition Cookbook*, Piatkus (2010)

Patrick Holford, *The Low-GL Diet Bible*, Piatkus (2009)

Patrick Holford and Fiona McDonald Joyce, *The Low-GL Diet Cookbook*, Piatkus (2005)

Chapter 18

Patrick Holford et al., *How to Quit Without Feeling S**t*, Piatkus (2008)

Chapter 20

Stephanie Merritt, *The Devil Within*, Vermilion (2009)

RESOURCES

The Brain Bio Centre is the clinic of the Food for the Brain Foundation in Richmond, on the outskirts of London. It specialises in the Optimum Nutrition approach to mental health, under the direction of Patrick Holford. The Centre's team works with clients to identify any nutritional or biochemical imbalances that may be contributing to their symptoms and provides a tailored programme to correct these issues and restore health. Through a process of nutritional and psychiatric assessment, appropriate clinical tests, dietary advice and/or supplements will then be recommended. Visit www.brainbiocentre.com, address: Avalon House, 72 Lower Mortlake Road, Richmond, TW9 2JY, UK, tel.: +44 (0)20 8332 9600

The Food for the Brain Foundation is a non-profit educational organisation directed by Patrick Holford, which aims to promote awareness of the link between learning, behaviour, mental health and nutrition, and to educate and provide educational material to children, parents, teachers, schools, the public, the catering industry, health professionals and the government. The website contains useful information on nutrition, depression and mental-health issues. For more information visit www.foodforthebrain.org; tel.: +44 (0)20 8788 3801

The Institute for Optimum Nutrition (ION) offers a three-year foundation degree course in nutritional therapy, which includes training in the optimum nutrition approach to mental health. Visit www.ion. ac.uk, address: Avalon House, 72 Lower Mortlake Road, Richmond, TW9 2JY, UK; tel.: +44 (0)20 8332 9600

Nutritional therapy and consultations To find a nutritional therapist near you whom I recommend, visit www.patrickholford.com. This service gives details on who to see in the UK as well as internationally.

If there is no one available near you, you can always take an on-line assessment – see below.

Online 100% Health Programme Are you 100 per cent healthy? Find out with our FREE health check and comprehensive personalised 100% Health Programme, giving you a personalised action plan, including diet and supplements. Visit www.patrickholford.com.

Zest4Life is a health and nutrition club, based on low-GL principles, that provides advice, coaching and support for losing weight and gaining health through a series of weekly meetings. There are also groups that focus specifically on improving mood. For more information, visit www.zest4life.eu.

Psychocalisthenics is an excellent exercise system that takes less than 20 minutes a day, and develops strength, suppleness and stamina as well as generating vital energy. The best way to learn it is to do the Psychocalisthenics Training. See www.patrickholford.com (events) for details. Also available is the book *Master Level Exercise: Psychocalisthenics* and the *Psychocalisthenics* CD and DVD from www. patrickholford.com (shop). For further information on pcals please see www.pcals.com.

Silence of Peace (CD) Based on centuries-old use of specific musical scales and arrangements, the music CDs of John Levine help you to enter a more relaxed and peaceful state of mind. Suitable for both adults and children. To find out more and purchase, visit www.patrickholford. com.

Meditative CDs that very specifically change your brainwave patterns into a mindful state (alpha and theta waves) and away from negative thought patterns are highly effective for some people. Visit www. patrickholford.com/meditation to find out more.

Psychotherapy To find a psychotherapist or counsellor in your area, contact the United Kingdom Council for Psychotherapy. Visit www. psychotherapy.org.uk; tel.: 020 7014 9955; email: info@ukcp.org.uk.

I have been particularly impressed by psychotherapists and counsellors trained at the Psychosynthesis and Education Trust, 92–94 Tooley Street, London Bridge, London SE1 2TH. They also have an excellent workshop called The Essentials that enables you to look at your life, how you would like it to be and what needs to change. The Essentials is run either as a five-day intensive programme or over two long weekends. Visit www.psychosynthesis.edu/; tel.: 020 7403 2100; email: enquiries@petrust.org.uk.

The Hoffman Process is an eight-day intensive residential course in which you are shown how to let go of the past, release pent-up stress, self-limiting behaviours and resentments, and start creating the future you desire. Visit www.hoffmaninstitute.co.uk, address Box 72, Quay House, River Road, Arundel, West Sussex, BN18 9DF; tel.: 0800 068 7114 or +44 (0) 1903 889 990; email: info@hoffmaninstitute.co.uk. Courses are also offered in South Africa, Australia, Singapore and other parts of the world. For details on these and other international centres visit www.hoffmaninstitute.com.

Human Givens You may find this helpful, especially if you are waking up tired, exhausted and depressed. The Human Givens approach provides a holistic, scientific framework for understanding the way that individuals and society work. It encompasses the latest scientific understanding from neurobiology and psychology, as well as ancient wisdom and original new insights. See www.humangivens.com for products and details of seminars/workshops.

Support with thyroid problems The best place to find a list of sympathetic doctors is through one of these two patient support groups: Thyroid Patient Advocacy-UK: www.tpa-uk.org.uk; Thyroid UK: www.thyroiduk.org.

The Sleep Assessment Advisory Service helps people who are suffering from insomnia. Tel.: 028 9262 2266.

Laboratory tests

Food Allergy (IgG ELISA), homocysteine, GLCheck (which measures your level of glycosylated haemoglobin, also called HbA1C) and Livercheck tests are available through YorkTest Laboratories, using a home test kit. You take your own pinprick blood sample and return it to the lab for analysis. Visit www.yorktest.com, or call freephone (UK) 0800 074 6185. These test kits are also available from www.totallynourish.com.

Tests for serotonin and noradrenalin levels are available from the Brain Bio Centre for its patients. Visit www.foodforthebrain.org.

Intestinal permeability (leaky gut) test This test is available from the following labs through qualified nutrition consultants and doctors:

Biolab Medical Unit (doctor's referral only): visit www.biolab.co.uk; tel.: +44 (0)20 7636 5959/5905.
Genova Diagnostics: visit www.gdx.uk.net; tel.: +44 (0)20 8336 7750.

Andropause You can test your symptoms and also get a salivary testosterone test by visiting www.andropause.com.

Genetic testing is available from www.genetic-health.co.uk.

Health products

Xylitol The low-GL natural sugar alternative, xylitol, is available from health-food shops and from www.totallynourish.com.

Cherry Active is sold in a highly concentrated juice format. Mix a 30ml (2 tbsp) serving with 250ml (9fl oz) water to make a deliciously healthy, low-GL cherry juice. Each 946ml bottle contains the juice from over 3,000 cherries – that's half a tree's worth – and contains a month's supply. Cherry Active is also available as a dried cherry snack and in capsules. For more information and to order, visit www.totallynourish.com (see page 253).

Chia seeds, the highest vegetarian source of omega 3, are also available from www.totallynourish.com.

Full-spectrum lighting works by duplicating the light from the sun and has several associated health benefits such as relief from seasonal affective disorder, improved mood, better mental alertness, regulated sleep and increased vitamin D absorption. For full-spectrum light bulbs, reading lights and 'dawn alarm' clocks visit www.sad.uk.com.

Supplements and suppliers

Finding your own perfect supplement programme can be confusing, but my website, www.patrickholford.com, offers useful guidance.

The backbone of a good supplement programme is:

- A high strength multivitamin
- Additional vitamin C, including other synergistic immune-boosting nutrients
- An essential fat supplement containing omega-3 and omega-6 oils

In this section are examples of supplements that provide the herbs and nutrients at the levels discussed in this book. The addresses of the companies whose products I've referred to are given at the end.

Multivitamin and mineral supplements

Supplementing the right multivitamin is the most important supplement decision you make. Most multis are based on RDA levels of nutrients, which are not the same as optimum nutrition levels. A good multivitamin based on optimum nutrition levels is BioCare's Optimum Nutrition Formula. Another is Solgar's VM2000. Both of these recommend taking two tablets a day. Optimum Nutrition Formula has higher mineral levels, especially for calcium and magnesium. Ideally, take a multivitamin and mineral with an extra 1g of vitamin C. BioCare's Optimum Nutrition Pack provides the multivitamin, extra vitamin C and essential omega-3 and -6 oils all in a daily strip.

Essential fats and fish oil supplements

The most important omega-3 fats are DHA, DPA and EPA, both in oily fish and in cod liver oil. The most important omega-6 fat is GLA, the richest source being borage (also known as starflower) oil. Try BioCare's Essential Omegas, which provide a highly concentrated mix of EPA, DHA, DPA and GLA. They also produce Mega-EPA, a high-potency omega-3 fish oil supplement. Seven Seas produce Extra High Strength Cod Liver Oil.

Digestive enzymes and support

A good digestive enzyme combination should contain protease, amylase and lipase, which digest protein, carbohydrate and fat respectively. Some also contain amyloglucosidase (helps to digest glucosides found in certain beans and vegetables) and lactase (helps to digest milk sugars). If you get bloated after lentils or beans, such as soya products, choose an enzyme that contains alpha-galactosidase. Try Solgar's Vegan Digestive Enzymes. You can also buy digestive enzymes *with* probiotics: BioCare's DigestPro contains all these enzymes and probiotics.

Probiotics/digestive enzymes/gut repair

Probiotics are supplements of beneficial bacteria, the two main strains being *Lactobacillus acidophilus* and *Bifidobacterium bifidus*. There are various types of strains within these two, some more important in children, others in adults. There is quite some variability in amounts of bacteria (some labels say things like 'a billion viable organisms per capsule') and quality. A very good product is BioCare's Bio-Acidophilus and also DigestPro, which also contains digestive enzymes and glutamine.

Methyl nutrient/homocysteine complexes

A good methyl nutrient complex should contain at least vitamins B_6, B_{12} and folic acid. Some formulas also contain vitamin B_2, trimethylglycine (TMG), zinc, and N-acetyl-cysteine. Three products that fulfil this criteria are BioCare's Connect, which contains them all; Solgar's Gold Specifics Homocysteine Modulators, which contain TMG, vitamins B_6, B_{12} and folic acid; or Higher Nature's 'H Factors', which contain vitamins B_2, B_6, B_{12}, folic acid and zinc, plus TMG (see www.highernature.co.uk).

Mood support nutrients

BioCare offer a comprehensive range of nutritional combination packs to address specific needs and deficiencies as highlighted in this book.

Awake Food is designed to support the body's level of alertness and feelings of energy. As well as vitamins B_5, B_6 and B_{12}, it also contains tyrosine, the amino acid which acts as a precursor to the neurotransmitter dopamine, and the hormone thyroxine. Brain Food contains nutrients for neurotransmitter reception and production, including phosphatidylcholine and DMAE, B_{12}, folic acid and pantothenic acid.

Chill Food is a blend of vitamins, amino acids and plant extracts to support the body's nervous system and help promote healthy levels of sleep. It contains taurine and 5-HTP, together with magnesium and vitamins B_6, B_{12}, folic acid and pantothenic acid. Mood Food contains both 5-HTP and tyrosine to support the body's production of important 'feel good' brain neurotransmitters as well as co-factor B vitamins to help support neurotransmitter production and balance, vitamin D and chromium.

St John's wort

This herb can be taken in tablet form, but it is often available as a tincture that can be added to water or juice. Solgar and Viridian are brands to look for in a good health store. A herbalist can also make up a tincture for you.

Thyroid support

The amino acid tyrosine is key to supporting good thyroid function. An ideal way to take it is in a combination formula that includes the other nutrients needed to support its conversion into throxine. BioCare's Awake Food is an excellent option. Also, kelp tablets are a rich source of iodine, needed for the healthy function of the thyroid, and can be picked up in all good health stores.

Vitamin D

This vitamin can be purchased easily from health stores from suppliers including Higher Nature, Viridian and Solgar. For quick absorption, you might want to consider sublingual (under the tongue) drops from BioCare.

Sugar balance

Look for a supplement that contains 200mcg of chromium, either as chromium polynicotinate or chromium picolinate, ideally with cinnamon high in MCHP. (Cinnulin PF is the name of a concentrated extract of cinnamon that is especially high in MCHP.)

Skincare products

Environ products were developed by the cosmetic surgeon Dr Des Fernandes to prevent skin cancer and address the damaging effects of the environment on our skin. Formulated with scientifically proven active ingredients, including vitamin A and antioxidant vitamins C, E and beta-carotene, which are used in progressively higher concentrations, Environ will maintain a normal healthy skin or effectively treat and prevent the signs of ageing, pigmentation, problem skin and scarring. Environ products are available from www.totallynourish.com or direct from an Environ skincare therapist. See www.vitaminskincare.eu to find one near you in the EU. For international enquiries call +27 21 683 1034 or email environc@africa.com, or visit www.environ.co.za.

Supplement suppliers

The following companies produce good-quality supplements that are widely available in the UK.

BioCare offers an extensive range of nutritional and herbal supplements, including daily 'packs', which are good for travelling/when you are away from home. Their products are stocked by most good health-food stores. Visit www.biocare.co.uk; tel.: +44 (0)121 433 3727. They are also available by mail order from Totally Nourish (www.totallynourish.com) – see below.

Higher Nature Available from most independent health-food stores or visit www.highernature.co.uk; tel.: 0800 458 4747.

Solgar Available in most independent health-food stores or visit www.solgar-vitamins.co.uk; tel.: +44 (0) 1442 890355.

Viridian For stockists visit www.viridian-nutrition.com; tel.: +44 (0) 1327 878050

Totally Nourish is an 'ɛ'-health shop that stocks many high-quality health products, including home test kits and supplements. Visit www. totallynourish.com; tel.: 0800 085 7749 (freephone within the UK).

And in other regions:

South Africa

The original PATRICK HOLFORD vitamin and supplement brand from the UK is now available in South Africa through leading health food shops, Dis-Chem, and Clicks retail pharmacies. They are also available on-line direct from www.holforddirect.co.za by post or by courier direct to your door. PATRICK HOLFORD supplements, books and CDs can also be ordered by phone on 011 2654 554.

Australia

Solgar supplements are available in Australia. Visit www.solgar.com. au; tel.: 1800 029 871 (free call) for your nearest supplier. Another good brand is Blackmores.

New Zealand

BioCare products (see opposite) are available in New Zealand through Aurora Natural Therapies. Visit www.Aurora.org.nz, address:12a Battys Road, Springlands, Blenheim 7201, New Zealand.

Singapore

BioCare (see opposite) and Solgar products are available in Singapore through Essential Living. Visit www.essliv.com; tel.: 6276 1380.

UAE

BioCare supplements (see opposite) are available in Dubai from Organic Foods & Café, P.O. Box 117629, Dubai, United Arab Emirates; tel.: +971 44340577; fax.: +971 44340577.

INDEX

Note: Page numbers in **bold** refer to diagrams.

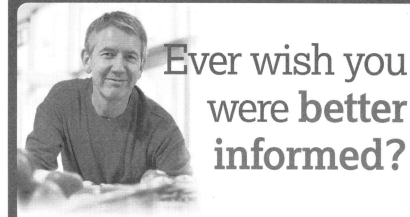

Ever wish you were better informed?

Join my 100% Health Club today and you'll receive:

✔ My newsletter, plus Special Reports on vital health topics.

✔ Immediate access to hundreds of health articles and special reports.

✔ Have your questions answered in our Members Only blogs.

✔ Save money on supplements, books and other health products.

✔ Save up to £50 on Patrick Holford's **100% Health Workshop**.

✔ Become part of a community of like-minded people and help others.

JOIN TODAY at www.patrickholford.com

❝ Being a member has transformed my life, and that of many of my family and friends. Patrick's information is always spot on and really practical. My member benefits and discounts save me much more than the subscription. Being a member is a must if you want to be and stay healthy. ❞

Joyce Taylor

100%Health®
Weekend Intensive
The workshop that works.

D	C	B	A
NOT GOOD	AVERAGE	REASONABLY HEALTHY	SUPER HEALTHY
	Karen before: 36%		Karen after: 86%

Learn how to go from 'average' to superhealthy in a weekend.

Do YOU want to:

✔ Take control of your own health?

✔ Master your weight?

✔ Turn back the clock?

✔ Prevent and reverse disease?

✔ Transform your diet, your health and your life?

Discover the **8 secrets of optimum living** - and put them into action with your own individualised personal health and fitness programme with **Patrick Holford**.

"I thought I was healthy. I feel absolutely fantastic. It's changed my life." Karen S.

"Learnt more in a day than a lifetime. Definitely recommended." Sarah F.

"It worked miraculously. I lost 5 stones in 5 months. Life has become very good." Fiona F.

"I have so much more energy. I wake up raring to go. It's changed my life." Matthew F.

"You can wake up full of energy, with a clear mind and balanced mood, never gain weight and stay disease free. Having worked with over 60,000 people I know what changes are going to most rapidly transform how you feel."
Patrick Holford

"Visionary." *Independent*

"Health guru Patrick Holford addresses the true causes of illness." *Guardian*

"One of the world's leading authorities on new approaches to health" *Daily Mail*

Thousands of people have transformed their health.
Why not become one of them?
For more information see **www.patrickholford.com**

100%Health® is the registered trademark of Holford & Associates